Toxic Electricity

© Copyright: Steven Magee 2012

Edition 2 - 2013

Cover Picture: Electrical emissions have changed the electromagnetic radiation (EMR) transmission from the Sun to the ground.

Contents

Introduction

The modern electrical system was invented by Nikola Tesla. While acknowledged as one of his greatest achievements, there is a side of Nikola Tesla that many people do not know. In the first half of his life he was a brilliant man. However, for the second half of his life he was widely acknowledged as being mentally ill. As such, Toxic Electricity investigates the problems with the modern electrical system and how it can affect human health.

Electrical systems have been shown time and time again to increase the risk of human illness and disease. Mental illness is one of these diseases and it is not surprising to see the inventor of the alternating current (AC) electricity system develop it. What is surprising is that over one hundred years after the invention of AC electricity that the detrimental health effects of AC electricity are still in denial by many governments, corporations, utilities, and health and safety organizations.

Rather than acknowledge the health issues and develop research into the toxic effects of AC electricity, the opposite has happened. AC electricity health research is almost none existent and the development of the AC electrical power system is rampant around the world. Billions of dollars pour into the development of AC electricity annually in the USA alone.

"There is a cult of ignorance in the United States, and there has always been. The strain of anti-intellectualism

*has been a constant thread winding its way through our
political and cultural life, nurtured by the false notion that
democracy means that "my ignorance is just as good as
your knowledge." - Isaac Asimov*

The electrical system has been changing since the days of
Nikola Tesla. It is a system that has been significantly
altered by the advent of the electronics industry. Electronic
power generation and electronic devices are in the process
of changing the way the electrical system works.
Harmonics is a poorly understood aspect of electrical
engineering and is a characteristic feature of electronics.
Harmonics greatly increases the electromagnetic radiation
emissions from the electrical system and my research is
indicating that it causes biological damage and mutations.

If you own electronic products, then your home and work
place may be filled with harmonic energy fields!

The effects of harmonic energy are added to by the
development of wireless communications. Today, there are
fields of energy in your environment that have never
existed in the history of the human and we will investigate
the impacts on human health. Did you know that there are
human sickness "Hot Zones" around cell phone towers? If
you are feeling tired, it may be the cell phone tower near
your home that is interfering with your energy levels.

Electrical lighting products seem harmless, but may
actually be inducing a myriad of illnesses into the human,
and that includes cancer! The lighting products that are
available today vary widely. We will review them and
advise on the safest forms of these products for the human

environment. This is particularly important if you have babies and developing children in your home.

A concerning development is that approximately 300,000 people in Sweden have registered as having Electromagnetic Hypersensitivity (EHS). EHS is caused by exposure to electrical, electronic and wireless products and Sweden is the only country that currently recognizes it as a health condition. This new epidemic in the population is predicted to keep on increasing as the use of technology gains momentum.

We will discuss the various aspects of the electrical system throughout the book and take a look at how the march of electronics into the electrical system has caused it to change. Electricity has been known to be a factor in many illnesses and diseases and we are now in an era of the modern electrical system that this rate and range of illness and disease is increasing.

Diagrams and photographs are used to illustrate many of the concepts of the book. If you are reading this in black and white, then descriptions of the pictures accompany them to explain the concepts. The concepts of the book should be accessible to most people through the visual explanations of subjects discussed in the book. Key points will be in bold font.

This book is aimed at the general public, the medical profession and the engineering profession. Extensive mathematics is avoided and the book presents the health concepts of the modern electrical system in a readable format to the general public.

This book contains the very latest research on the human environment. It should be viewed as the current ideas on the subject and the contents are subject to review by the scientific community.

The author and publisher accept no liability whatsoever for any of the contents and the book is published in the spirit of unrestricted access to the latest ideas and scientific theories in a changing world.

You should always consult with a licensed and certified medical professional on any aspects of health, illness or disease.

"It's a rare person who wants to hear what he doesn't want to hear."

Dick Cavett

Electricity

This quote is a good summary of what has happened in the last 100 years:

"All life on Earth has adapted to survive in an environment of weak, natural low-frequency electromagnetic fields (in addition to the Earth's static geomagnetic field). Natural low-frequency EM fields come from 2 main sources: the Sun and thunderstorm activity. But in the last one hundred years, man-made fields at much higher intensities and with a very different spectral distribution have altered this natural EM background in ways that aren't yet fully understood." - Unknown.

We have all been born into an electrical society. Today, there is no place on Earth that is free of man-made electromagnetic radiation with the advent of ground based radio and microwave transmissions and later, Space satellites that are routinely beaming electromagnetic energy to the surface of the Earth.

I was born in 1970 in Europe and I have never experienced life free from electricity. Electricity has always been close by wherever I have traveled in life. Like most people, I never really thought about the detrimental health aspects of it. It is the same with light. The presence of electric lighting has just been a normal part of life for me. No one ever told me it was harmful.

It is also the same with the Sun. No one really educated me about it. My behavior around sunlight revolved around not getting burned and enjoying sunny days.

Sunlight, artificial light, and electricity are all part of the electromagnetic radiation spectrum and this is shown on the next page.

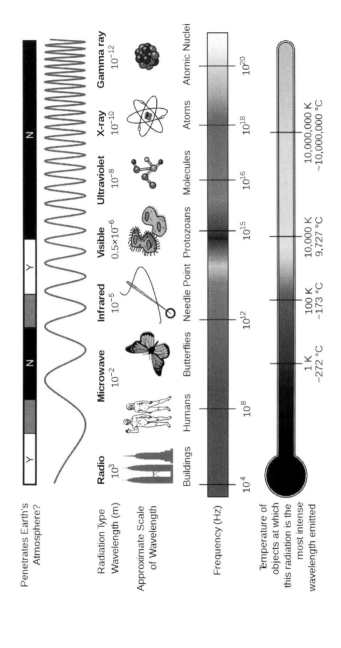

With the advent of radio and microwave communication technologies, our environment is now filled with electrical energy. You are now subjected to a wide range of man-made electromagnetic frequencies that were not there just a few decades ago. Indeed the man-made electromagnetic spectrum is increasing on a daily basis as the human addiction to modern technologies continues to gain momentum.

As the use of technology is increasing, we are witnessing the rise of childhood development problems, human illness, cancer, and the shortening of the human lifespan. They are all connected and it would be foolish to ignore this fact. Indeed, in 2011 the link between cancer and cellphones has become established. Cellphones in the future may be viewed the same way that asbestos and cigarettes are today.

Aside from the soup of man-made electromagnetic radiation that we now find ourselves immersed into, we have changed the atmospheric gas composition drastically over the last few hundred years of the Industrial Revolution. This is commonly referred to by many as the carbon levels rising in the atmosphere. They are currently at double the recorded levels in the historical records and there are no doubts that the use of energy to fuel the Industrial Revolution caused this to occur.

This is changing the natural electromagnetic environment that nature produces. Human actions are changing the energy fields that we are walking around in. The most unnatural electromagnetic environments are found in the home and workplace. It is quite possible that your home may actually be the most toxic place that you spend time in.

It is hard to believe that your home may be toxic to you, but it is true. While the toxicity of homes is extensive, we will stay in the area of electromagnetic radiation exposures in this book.

Homes started to get really toxic with electromagnetic radiation exposures when the building codes required an electrical socket to be installed every ten feet in the home. Take a look around you, you are never far from an electrical outlet. That also means that you are never far from an AC electrical cable.

When you are in a room in your home, you have an AC voltage waveform riding on your body. I first noticed this effect when I was sixteen and working with oscilloscopes at the engineering training center. It looks just like the AC waveform on the electrical cables, just a lower voltage. This is shown in the next picture.

The human body has a voltage waveform riding on it when near to AC electricity. This waveform reduces the further away you get from the electrical system.

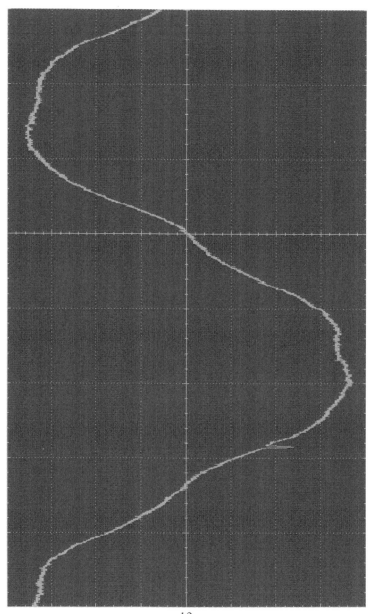

Everyone told me that it was harmless when I noticed it when I was sixteen. The problem is, it is not harmless!

To understand some of the things that the book talks about, we need to introduce some terms that are used in electrical engineering:

- Most electrical research has been done on pure 50Hz and 60Hz electrical sine waves. Hertz (Hz) is a measurement of frequency. It basically is the number of sine waves per second. The American electricity system is 60Hz and that means that there are 60 sine waves per second on the electrical cables.

- It is called an alternating current (AC) system due to the first half of the sine wave being positive polarity and the second half of the sine wave being negative. So the AC electrical current is constantly reversing many times per second, hence the term "alternating".

- Electrical current (I) on the system only flows when you plug something in or turn something on. This is called the "impedance" (load) and the current that flows on the system will be dependent on the impedance. Electrical current is analogous to the speed of a flowing river.

- The voltage (V) is the potential difference between two points. The higher the voltage is, the more energy you can send through an electrical cable. Contact with voltage is considered dangerous to a dry human at above 50 volts and may cause electrocution to occur. Electrical voltage is analogous to the width of a river.

- Watts (W) is a measurement of electrical energy and is obtained simply by multiplying the voltage with the current. It is analogous to the surface area of water flowing in a river.

- Impedance (Ohm) is used to control the flow of electrical current. It is analogous to the slope of the river. High impedance would be similar to a level river that has a very slow flow. Low impedance would be akin to a fast flowing river on a steep slope.

- An electrical short circuit would be comparable to the fastest flow of water that occurs. Short circuits are what blow the fuse or trip the circuit breaker. This is akin to a dam bursting and creating a very high flow of water in the river. This high flow is prevented by using fuses or circuit breakers that stop the flow a short time after the dam busts.

- Electromagnetic fields are produced by the various forms of electricity and they have two components to them. These are electric and magnetic fields. The electric field is a result of the voltage and the magnetic field is produce by the current flow. The higher the current and voltage are, the higher the electromagnetic fields become.

- Electromagnetic interference (EMI) is caused by the presence of man-made electromagnetic fields that expose the human to unnatural electromagnetic radiation that it has no genetic adaptation to.

There is a problem with performing research on a pure AC sine wave because that is not how the system works in real life. In the real world of AC electricity there are many higher frequencies of energy on the system. This has become especially apparent with the adoption of electronics because the loads on the system add frequencies of energy to the system.

This real world AC electricity is termed "Dirty Electricity" and it is very harmful to the human. Dirty electricity puts very large fields onto cables and may completely fill your home with electromagnetic radiation fields. The people who are most vulnerable to the effects of this are babies and young children. Attention Deficit Disorder (ADD) and Autism are on the rise and may well be connected to the effects of dirty electricity.

Samuel Milham, MD, MPH, has researched this area and has found from census data that many illnesses and diseases were born with the adoption of electricity into the home and workplace. His book "Dirty Electricity" extensively documents his findings in this area.

It is not just the electricity that is causing health problems in the general population, it is also the products that the electricity powers. You may be purchasing products that are making your family sick and not even realize it! Certain combinations of products when connected to your electrical system can make it start to radiate large electromagnetic fields into your environment.

The human mind and body cannot sense most forms of electromagnetic radiation. It shows up as general sickness that may move onto disease and perhaps premature death. As such, it is important to be aware of your electromagnetic environment.

We will start by looking into the most common application of electricity and that is light.

"Natural electromagnetic relationships form the basis of all cycles in nature. The construction and preservation of these relationships is only possible due to natural energy and their destruction takes place because of energy emanating from the technological unnatural energy"

Hertel

Electric Light

Electric light presents a hazard to human health. There are many sources of electric light and you should learn to recognize these sources. Electric light is almost everywhere in modern society:

- Artificial street lighting.
- Artificial home lighting.
- Artificial office lighting.
- Car headlights.
- Traffic lights.
- Signs.
- Emergency vehicle lights.
- Security lights.
- Televisions of every type.
- Computer monitors of every type.

So what may electric light be shown to do in the future? In the future the following conditions may be proven to be related to electric light:

- Cancer.
- Depression.
- Heart attacks.
- Circulation issues.

- Diabetes.
- Brain and nerve issues.
- Disruption of circadian rhythm.
- General aches and pains.
- Aggression.
- Psychiatric problems.
- Gender changing.
- Triggering of the mating cycle.
- Increased fertility.
- Conception issues.
- Sexual dysfunction.
- Almost any of the current medical problems in society may be related to electric light.

Dr. John Nash Ott was the leading researcher in this field and he had extensively proven that he could induce cancer, brain disease, sleep problems, aggression, and gender changing into plants and animals by the end of the 1980's. He did this simply by exposing them to electrical lighting products!

The problems with the particular types of electric light are as follows:

- Artificial light:
  - Artificial lighting is not full spectrum daylight and may cause illness in the human body.
- Office lighting:

- This tends to be florescent lighting and is produced by just a few colors of light. It has a very spiked spectrum which does not occur in nature. The electronics that control them may emit electromagnetic interference (EMI).

- TV and computer monitors:

  - These tend to produce their light by mixing red, green and blue colors and it is an unusual spectrum which does not occur in nature. The light is similar to florescent lights. The electronics that control them may emit electromagnetic interference (EMI).

- Street lights:

  - Street lights are predominantly gas discharge lighting and this is one of the most toxic forms of lighting to the human mind and body. The light tends to be monochromatic and they have problems with emitting electromagnetic interference (EMI).

- Neon signs:

  - These tend to have similar problems as streetlights.

You should be careful when choosing a home to live in and pay close attention to the location of streetlights. Streetlights can emit large amounts of electromagnetic radiation, especially so when they switch on and also when they start to fail. The light also tends to be monochromatic or have a spiked spectrum of light and this type of light was shown by Dr. John Nash Ott to be harmful to the human mind and body. Indeed, I have noticed a trend in people who have died prematurely young and the presence of streetlights outside of their properties.

Regarding the toxic effects of lighting, I found during a Dieffenbachia plant growth experiment in my home that I started to get ill with fatigue, headaches, and insomnia. The experiment was performed by growing plants under the following light sources: Light emitting diode (LED), compact florescent (CFL), and a high pressure sodium street light (SOX).

After two weeks I decided to discontinue the experiment and within a day I had noticed withdrawal symptoms showing up that cleared up within the space of three days. This comprised of aches and pains in my feet, legs, chest, intestines, and head. On the second day of withdrawal a large headache appeared that would not respond to medication and this lasted for two days. There were no doubts that this combination of products was the cause of the problems.

I had very little exposure to the light as they were in rooms that had their doors closed. Most of the time I was generally between 30 to 60 feet away from the products. The products were switched on at 07:00 and turned off at 19:00 daily by automatic timers. I would check the experiment in the morning to ensure that the lights had turned on and in the evening to ensure that the lights had turned off.

My conclusion is that extended exposure to the electromagnetic radiation that this combination of

lighting products produced was sufficient to produce depression symptoms into the human.

The streetlight exposed plant died several months later. The CFL and LED plants went on to show strange stunted growth patterns with very small glossy dark green leaves.

The diagrams on the following pages show the various electric lighting effects. Electromagnetic interference, harmonics and stray voltage/current/frequency will be looked into later in the book.

Streetlight Emissions

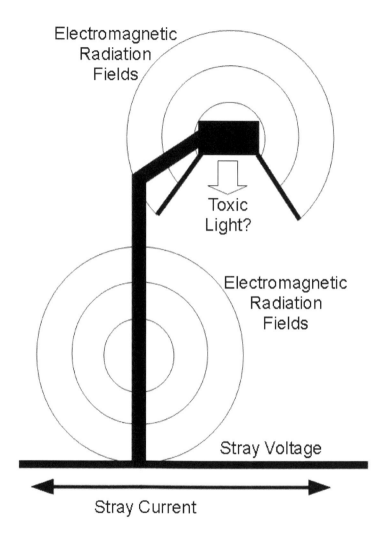

Three light bulbs are shown. At the top is the high pressure sodium light (SOX), the middle shows the compact florescent light (CFL), and the bottom shows the light emitting diode (LED) light.

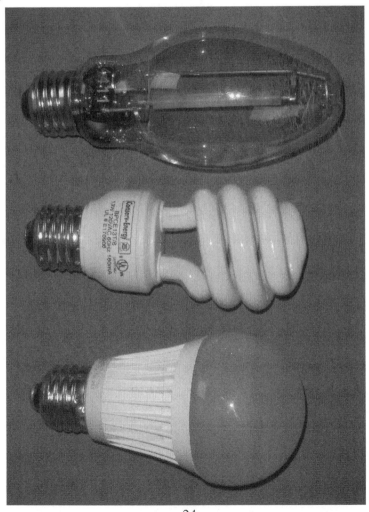

This is the current waveform for the three products combined. Note the distortion in the sine wave.

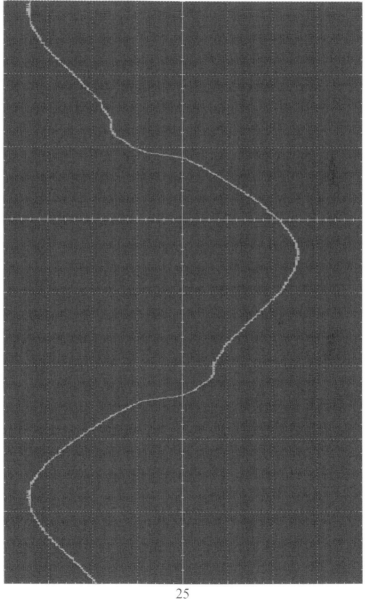

This is the frequency content of the current waveform for the combined three products. The repeating spikes are known as the "Harmonics". Note that zero Hertz is at the bottom of the page and the highest frequency is at the top of the page for these frequency graphs.

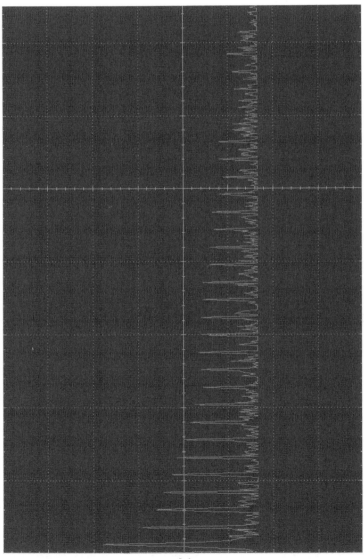

Dr. John Nash Ott called streetlights "Crime Lights" as he had noticed that in areas with them that the people would be subjected to higher rates of crime. This effect has been repeatedly shown to be true by other researchers in the field.

All types of artificial lighting have the possibility of making you ill. Artificial lighting should be avoided if your health is important to you.

I would recommend that you avoid the use of the new lighting that has been developed, such as gas discharge (florescent, sodium, mercury, neon, and so on) and light emitting diode (LED) lighting. These have been developed in order to use less energy at the expense of the quality of the light. They appear to create dirty electricity on your electrical system and large electromagnetic fields in your environment. They may turn your home wiring into a wide band radio transmitter!

In the case of the LED light, long term exposure to the semiconductor spectrum of light is currently unknown. The LED lights can be very bright and you may need to be careful that it does not damage your eyes in the long term. Certain types of LED lights are already acknowledged to be causing insomnia in people due to the large amount of blue light in their spectrum. Indeed, I noticed this effect when working with one. My sleep patterns were off for about two weeks after working with it.

When reviewing thestranger.com article "*Kill the Lights*", we find:

"The beams from the high-intensity, light-emitting diodes are striking. The rays turned my skin the color of white taffy and cast crisp shadows on the pavement. "Zombie blue" is exactly right: Like a day-for-night special effect in a vampire movie, the test streetlights create the sort of atmosphere where you almost expect the undead to emerge from the flower beds and begin eating your face."

A major problem with electronic lighting products such as florescent lights, compact florescent lights (CFL), and light emitting diode (LED) lights is that they use an electronic inverter system to control the lamp. The inverter system is built into electronic light bulbs. Inverter systems inject strange frequencies of energy back into the electrical system that they are connected to. So instead of having a 60 Hz electrical system, you actually have an electrical system that contains many far higher frequencies of energy. This significantly changes the electrical system and may have the ability to make you ill.

The electronic products also have what is known as a non-linear current draw. This means that they do not have a sinusoidal current draw, but rather a distorted current draw. This creates harmonics on the electrical system.

There are many people reporting health issues around compact florescent lights and it is probably linked to the high frequencies of electrical energies coupling into the human body. This is called "Biological Coupling" and we will look into this later in the book.

LED lights have not been around as long as CFL lights, so there are currently less reports of problems with these light bulbs. However, they are starting to emerge. The biological coupling effects of the LED light bulbs appear to be quite similar to the CFL.

My recommendation is to avoid these electronic forms of lighting products until more is known about their problems and how they can affect human health.

These effects can be seen in the following pictures.

This compact florescent light (CFL) draws current from the electrical system in spikes. It will put harmonics onto the electrical system.

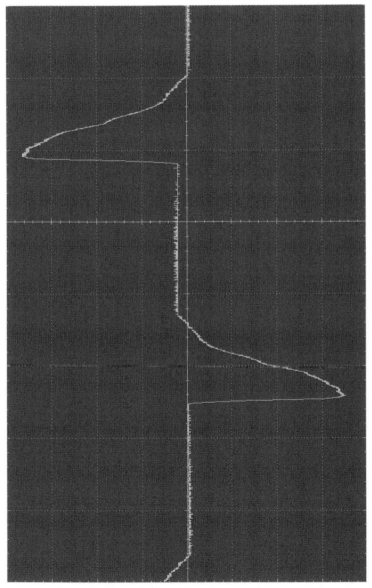

This is what the human body voltage looks like when near to it. There are a wide range of electrical energies on it.

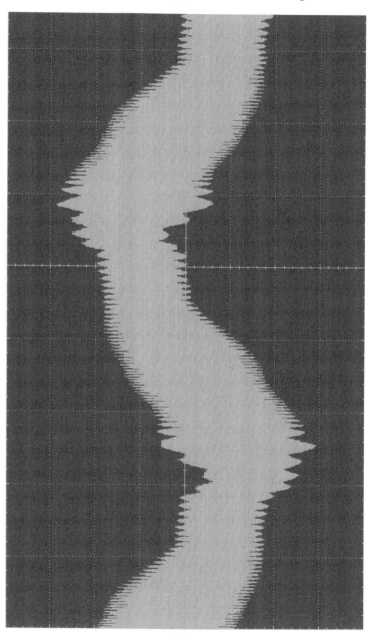

It has put a wide range of frequencies of electrical energy onto the human body, including a very large spike at 60,000 hertz.

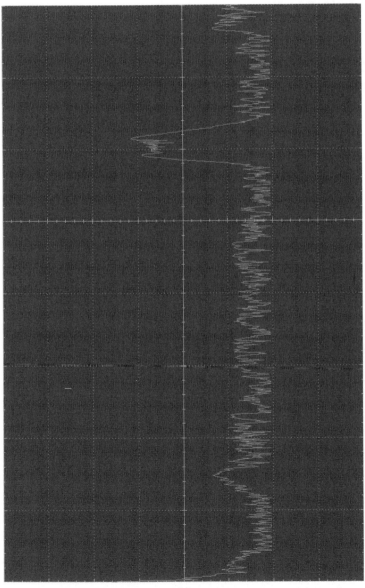

This is the current waveform for the light emitting diode (LED) light. It has a lot of distortion on it and this will create harmonics.

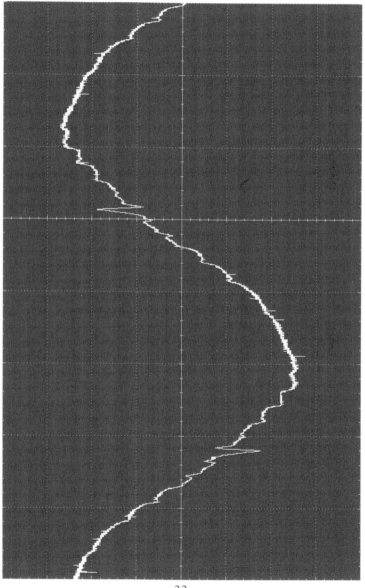

This is what the human body voltage looks like when near to it. There are many types of electrical energy.

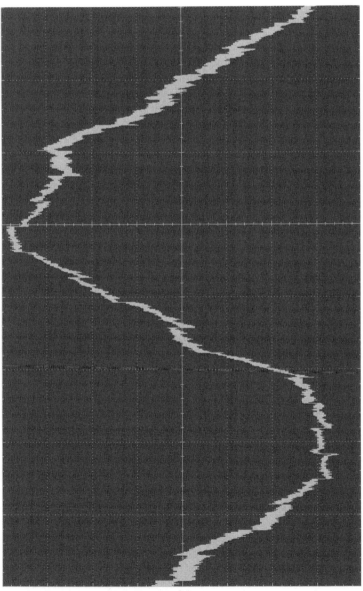

The human body voltage has a range of frequencies on it, including spikes at 62,500Hz, 125,000Hz and 187,500Hz.

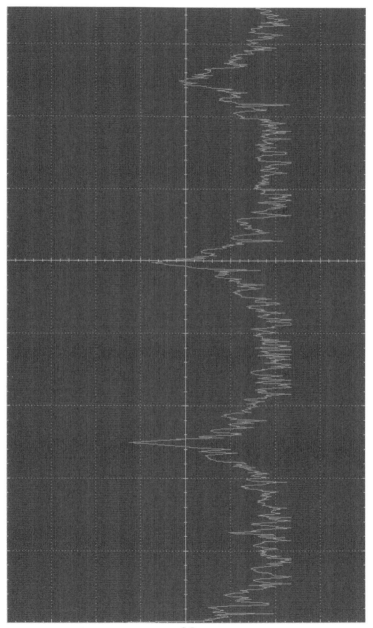

The newer LED lights may have a problem with longevity, particularly if installed into hot areas or enclosed light fittings. These are relatively new products and do not have a proven history of reliability yet.

People have formed a very unnatural habit of staring at computer screens for eight hours per day. This may have long term consequences for both your mental and physical health. You should avoid doing this and if your job requires it, then you should consider changing your job to one that does not require so much time in front of a computer. Computer generated light may changing how the mind works and there is much research being performed in this area currently. The long term health consequences of the latest generation of computer displays have yet to emerge. "Computer Vision Syndrome" is the medical term for the health effects that may occur from computer systems and some of the symptoms can be:

- Headaches.
- Blurred vision.
- Neck pain.
- Redness in the eyes.
- Fatigue.
- Eye strain.
- Dry eyes.
- Irritated eyes.
- Double vision.
- Polyopia.
- Difficulty refocusing the eyes.

The first edition of this book took me two weeks to write and had me working on a laptop computer with a 17 inch LED display for twelve hours per day. My previous exposure was about an hour per day. I had symptoms of tired eyes, irritated eyes, difficulty concentrating, and a withdrawal headache after I finished that was followed by tiredness. The week of proof reading the printed book and minor editing that followed was marked by dry, cracked and chapped lips that took weeks to clear up. There are no doubts that extended exposure to computer monitors can affect your health.

After having this experience, I later realized that it was preventable. Simply by moving the computer in front of a shady "full spectrum" window prevents the conditions from occurring. This is due to significantly diluting the artificial light from the computer monitor with outdoor light that the human is genetically adapted to. This is shown in the next picture.

It is likely that daytime office environments would be healthier if the ceiling was painted sky blue and the walls had green nature landscape scenes on them. Clearly, the office staff sitting facing shady full spectrum windows is already proven for its beneficial health effects and has been so for many decades. You should be aiming to keep your environment as natural as possible for good human health. Natural potted plants can assist in this process in the office environment.

Computer Screen Alignment

The correct alignment of a computer screen to the shaded full spectrum ultraviolet transmitting acrylic window.

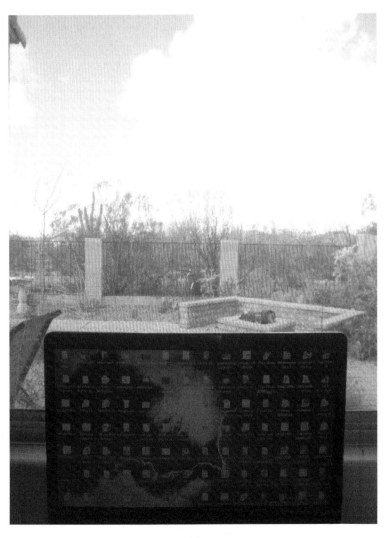

When reviewing the BBC News article *"Web addicts 'have brain changes'"*, we find:

"There was evidence of disruption to connections in nerve fibres linking brain areas involved in emotions, decision making, and self-control."

The recent adoption of large screen televisions may bring with it an increase in human health problems in the future. Large screen TV's consume a large amount of power and emit a corresponding amount of artificial light. Sitting too close to a large screen television may actually damage your health in the long term due to the excessive artificial light exposure from it. It is especially important to not let children sit close to the television for this reason.

Incorrect radiation levels may be able to affect your sex drive and it may be proven in the future that human sex drive is governed more by radiation types and levels than any other factor, even more so than hormones! Generally, a feeling of contentment replaces sexual desire in natural radiation environments.

There are many differences in the colors and spectrums of lighting products and each type of light may be able to affect you in a certain way. After much experimentation I have found that I prefer the light quality of soft white filament light bulbs for nighttime use.

You will only realize that the quality of light is bad when you contrast it to a known good light source. The standard to judge light by is outdoor daylight. There are no light bulbs that can match this standard and the closest thing that appears to do so is the halogen filament light bulb.

Most types of indoor lighting are known to be devoid of ultraviolet light (UV). This is a concern when used for daytime applications, as natural daytime UV light is essential to correct human development and good health. When reviewing the BBC News article *"Sun 'stops chickenpox spreading'"*, we find:

"UV light has long been known to inactivate viruses, and Dr Phil Rice, from St George's, University of London, who led the research, believes that this holds the key why chickenpox is less common and less easily passed from person to person in tropical countries."

The following photograph shows the difference between natural outdoor light and indoor light. The difference is striking!

Indoor light filtered by four panes of coated low-E glass on the left as contrasted to natural sunlight through an open window on the right. The center line is shade from the frame.

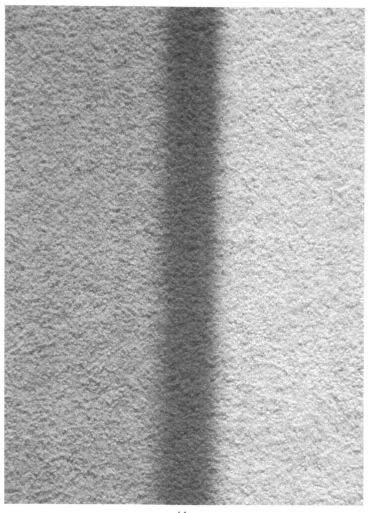

If you work in a daytime indoor environment, then the lighting should mimic what nature does. It should have a natural daytime spectrum of light that matches outdoor daylight. This would be achieved with full spectrum filament lights that have the correct amount of blue and ultraviolet light in their spectrums to mimic outdoor daylight. Your indoor lighting level should be approximately 1,000 lux (Lux is a measurement of brightness of light).

From 10:00 to 14:00 there should be an additional set of lights that is turned on that increases the brightness of the office environment, to mimic the peak in daylight that occurs outdoors. The indoor environment during this time should have an illumination level of approximately 2,000 lux. You can easily achieve this in your office environment by simply having a desk lamp that you switch on during that time to increase the light illumination that you are exposed to. You should be using full spectrum filament light bulbs of the correct spectral emissions for this exposure.

You should make sure that you go outdoors for an hour at solar noon and sit in the shade of trees. Do not wear any sunglasses, glasses, contacts, make-up nor sunscreen for this exposure. You need this exposure daily to keep up the solar cycle in the human mind and body. Without it, you may start to get fatigued as the day goes on. Daily outdoor exposure to sunlight is very important if you have an indoor occupation.

If you do not get the correct light exposures in the day, then your sleep cycle may kick in. The human body when kept in an indoor environment of low lux light

will not realize that it is daytime, as it cannot sense the increasing levels of daylight that the genetics are accustomed to. As such, by late morning your body may start sending a signal for you to sleep!

If you can, during any of your daily breaks, you should try and go outdoors to get natural daylight. You will also be getting fresh air and pollen exposure, which are also necessary for good health.

The recommended cycle for indoor daytime lighting is shown on the next page.

Indoor Daytime Lighting Cycle for Human Health

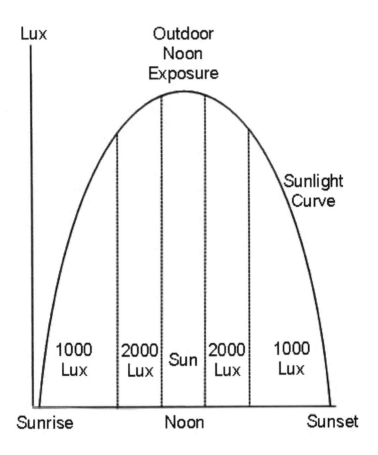

Nighttime lighting is very different from daytime lighting. You want to be using products that have minimal blue light in them. Blue light exposure is well known to cause insomnia. If you install lighting products that have too much blue light in their spectrums, then you may enter into a life of insomnia and not realize that it is your light bulbs that are causing it! Insomnia rapidly leads to fatigue and onto depression. These daytime lighting products are commonly sold as "Daylight" or "Full Spectrum" light bulbs and should not be used in nighttime applications.

You should stick to the tried and tested filament light bulbs for your nighttime exposures. Avoid the compact florescent and LED bulbs as some of these are well known for their excessive blue light content. Keep your lights low, as bright light can also trigger insomnia.

All electric lighting is unnatural and you should limit your exposure to it. Keep to lighting products that generate their light through heat and avoid products with unnaturally high amounts of blue light in them. These will appear excessively white to the eye and may induce insomnia into you. Filament lighting is the only lighting product that I advise people to use and keep the lighting levels low during the evening.

Low voltage halogen lighting products should be avoided due to the emissions from them. They may have high amounts of man-made ultraviolet light, some create dirty electricity, electric and magnetic fields. Man-made ultraviolet light is known for its ability to cause skin and eye problems and ultraviolet light is not present during the nighttime in nature. You will not find any electronic lamp dimmers in my home, as they are a product that you should avoid using. Lamp dimmers can create dirty electricity, electric and magnetic fields.

You should be using the correct voltage light bulb. In the USA these are sold as either 120 volt or 130 volt light bulbs. You should be using the 120 volt versions, as they are far more efficient at producing light. The 130 volt versions should only be used if your light bulbs are frequently breaking within a few days of installing them. If you use 130 volt light bulbs when they are not needed, your light bulbs will last a very long time, but will give out a poor quality of light.

You should be aware that the many sources of artificial lighting can affect your mental and physical health. You should be choosing your daytime artificial lighting products based on the proven health benefits of "Full Spectrum" light bulbs that are comparable to outdoor daylight. Health benefits have been reported by many gardeners who use these products to grow their plants indoors during the winter months. Nighttime artificial lighting products are different to daytime products and should be used in your home for good sleep patterns.

Nighttime over-illumination is a problem in the modern world and it may be able to affect your health. Keep it as low as possible during the nighttime and only increase lighting levels if you feel that you need more light in your environment. You should think candles, not necessarily use candles, but rather the illumination level that candles create. There is a reason why candles are considered romantic and it is likely related to the low level of light that they create.

If you have your environment too bright during the nighttime, then you may upset the circadian rhythm that governs your sleep cycles. Keep lighting as low as possible during the nighttime. You should also keep your skin covered as much as possible to prevent it from absorbing the artificial light.

Some lighting products suffer from flicker that is not noticeable to the eye. The newer LED lights and gas discharge lights appear to suffer from this effect. Indeed, most streetlights are actually flashing at 120 times per second. It is simply too fast for your eyes to detect it.

Flicker can do a lot of very strange things to the human mind and body. Commonly reported effects are:

- Epilepsy.
- Headaches.
- Disorientation.
- Anxiety.
- Seizures.
- Motion sickness.
- Eyestrain.

The health problems of flicker generally peak in the 5 to 30 times per second range. As such, you should not spend time in environments that have flashing or flickering lights. This may a problem for emergency service workers who work in environments that have these strobe lighting products in them. When multiple emergency vehicles are together, then their light flash rate will be much higher and may cause these problems to occur. The electromagnetic pulses from strobe lights may lead to electromagnetic hypersensitivity to occur in people who are close to them.

If you were to grow plants under strobe lighting products, you would notice a changed growth pattern. People have noticed that plants grow larger under them when compared to plants grown in a window. This is probably the plant reacting to the electromagnetic pulses and the high intensity light from the strobe. In nature, fast moving broken clouds can mimic the strobe lighting effect.

Many people say to mimic nighttime lighting by flame, as that is what we evolved in before the adoption of electricity. Both Dr. John Nash Ott and myself believe that it is healthier to go to bed when it goes dark and to avoid nighttime lighting of any kind. When reviewing the msnbc.com article *Nighttime lights linked to depression* we find:

"Exposure to a dim light at night, such as the glow of a TV screen, may prompt changes in the brain that lead to mood disorders, including depression, according to a new study in hamsters."

What lighting products do I have? I have conventional filament light bulbs at my home. You will not find any florescent, compact florescent (CFL), light emitting diode (LED), or any other types of lighting products within my home.

I use filament lighting products because they do not create dirty electricity effects on my home electrical system. I do not have any lamp dimmers. If I want the lighting levels lower, then I turn off some lights or use three way light bulbs.

There are extensive human mind and body photosynthesis effects taking place that react to light and for this reason it is important to understand the sensitivity of the human mind and body to light. Light in the human environment is an extensive subject that has many facets. As such, more information on light in the human environment can be found in the book "Toxic Light".

"Health and Light" by Dr. John Nash Ott is also recommended for further reading on this subject.

"Only a full spectrum of natural light could promote full health in plants, animals, and humans."

Dr. John Nash Ott.

Electromagnetic Radiation

"It is clear that radiation produces the electrical current which operates adaptively the organism as a whole, producing memory, reason, imagination, emotion, the special senses, secretions, muscular action, the response to infection, normal growth, and the growth of benign tumors and cancers, all of which are governed adaptively by the electric charges that are generated by the short wave or ionizing radiation in protoplasm."

Dr. George Crile.

Most people associate radiation with nuclear bombs, nuclear power plants, and X-ray machines. This is a very blinkered view and we will show you how extensive radiation in the human environment is and how critical it is for human health.

The modern human has created a radiation environment that has never existed before in all of human history and it keeps on adding to it every year. This is an issue as most of the sources of man-made radiation are not yet fully understood. As a radiation society, we are running before we have even learned to crawl!

The human radiation environment has many aspects to it:

- Solar radiation.
- Cosmic radiation.

- Environmental radiation.

Environmental radiation can come from many sources:

- Electrical storms.
- Static.
- Replacing nature with modern development significantly raises the levels of many types of radiation.
- Mining activities bring radioactive minerals to the surface which will increase the background radiation levels.
- Fall out from nuclear bombs and power plant disasters.
- Living close to a nuclear power station.
- Living close to a coal burning chimney.
- Living at altitude.
- Living near large bodies of water.
- Living in snowy climates.
- Living close to a military base.
- Living close to an airport or port.
- Living close to a hospital.
- Living close to any type of broadcast antenna.
- Living close to an amateur radio operator.
- Living close to power poles and lines.
- Living close to tall structures.
- Living close to glass covered buildings.

- Living in an area that is primarily concrete and asphalt.
- Being near to ionizing smoke detectors.
- Using transportation systems.
- Speed traps.
- Transmitting utility meters.
- Electrical products.
- Electronic products.
- Wireless devices.

Man-made electrical and electronic radiation did not exist until the 1800's when scientists started to discover the various forms of it. We have progressed extremely quickly from a new discovery to the many forms of it that are now present in modern society and this seems to have happened with little thought to the consequences to human health.

We now live in a society that is bombarded by electrical and electronic radiation. There is no place in the world that it does not reach with the prolific adoption of satellite and radio communications. Future historians will likely document this as one of the most foolish things that humanity ever did!

The electrical, electronic and wireless interference is commonly called:

- Electromagnetic Interference (EMI).
- Radio Frequency Interference (RFI).

- Microwave Frequency Interference (MFI).

For the purposes of this book we will use the term electromagnetic interference (EMI) for all of the above effects. The health effects of electromagnetic interference are commonly found documented as:

- Electromagnetic Hyper Sensitivity (EHS).
- Electro-Hyper-Sensitivity (EHS).
- Electrical Sensitivity (ES).
- Electro-Sensitivity (ES).
- Radio Wave Sickness (RWS).
- Rapid Aging Syndrome (RAS).
- Electrical Poisoning.
- Electronic Poisoning.
- Wireless Poisoning.
- Radiation Poisoning.
- Radiation Sickness.

For the purpose of this book, we will use the term electromagnetic hypersensitivity (EHS) to cover the above conditions. The strange thing about EHS is that many people have it, but very few of them realize that it is EHS that is causing their problems. EHS has not been publicized well and even many doctors do not appear to be aware of it. Strange, considering the amount of electrical, electronic and wireless equipment that we are now exposed to.

EHS is somewhat of an "Inconvenient Truth" and if it became widely accepted that it was causing human health problems, then many things would have to change. Industry and governments do not like change and in order to avoid it, it is far easier to deny it. For this reason, you should be aware of your environment and of EHS so that you can stay safe until it does become widely acknowledged as being the problem that it is.

The symptoms of it can be:

- Neurological:
    - Headaches.
    - Dizziness.
    - Nausea.
    - Difficulty concentrating.
    - Memory loss.
    - Irritability.
    - Dementia.
    - Depression.
    - Anxiety.
    - Insomnia.
    - Fatigue.
    - Weakness.
    - Tremors.
    - Numbness.
    - Tingling.

- Seizures.
- Paralysis.
- Psychosis.
- Stroke.
- Cardiac:
  - Palpitations.
  - Arrhythmia.
  - Pain or pressure in the chest.
  - Low or high blood pressure.
  - Slow or fast heart rate.
- Respiratory:
  - Shortness of breath.
  - Sinusitis.
  - Bronchitis.
  - Pneumonia.
  - Asthma.
  - Flu-like symptoms.
  - Fever.
- Dermatological:
  - Skin rash.
  - Itching.
  - Burning.
  - Facial flushing.
- Opthalmological:
  - Pain or burning in the eyes.

- ○ Pressure in or behind the eyes.
- ○ Deteriorating vision.
- ○ Floaters.
- ○ Cataracts.
- Muscular & Skeletal:
  - ○ Muscle spasms.
  - ○ Altered reflexes.
  - ○ Muscle and joint pain.
  - ○ Leg or foot pain.
  - ○ Arthritis.
  - ○ Swollen joints.
  - ○ Joint irritation.
- Others:
  - ○ Sexual problems.
  - ○ Digestive problems.
  - ○ Abdominal pain.
  - ○ Enlarged thyroid.
  - ○ Testicular or ovarian pain.
  - ○ Dryness of lips, tongue, mouth or eyes.
  - ○ Great thirst.
  - ○ Dehydration.
  - ○ Nose bleeds.
  - ○ Internal bleeding.
  - ○ Altered sugar metabolism.
  - ○ Immune abnormalities.

- Redistribution of metals within the body.
- Hair loss.
- Pain in the teeth.
- Deteriorating fillings.
- Impaired sense of smell.
- Ringing in the ears.
- Mouth ulcers.

Exposure to high frequencies may cause:

- Irregular heartbeat.
- Pains.
- Allergies.
- Miscarriages.
- Birth defects.
- Childhood leukemia.
- Brain tumors.
- Reproductive tumors.
- Cancers.
- Infertility.
- Depression.
- Chronic Fatigue Syndrome (CFS).
- Fibromyalgia.
- Gulf War Syndrome.
- Alzheimer's disease.

- Parkinson's disease.

- Lou Gehrig's disease.

- Behcet's Disease.

- Sexual arousal.

- Aggression.

Dr. Jim Burch PhD of the Cancer Prevention and Control Program at the University of South Carolina, has documented the biological effects of radio frequencies on the human mind and body as:

- **Cell proliferation (Increased ODC activity).**

- **Ion flux across biological membranes (Ca^{++}).**

- **DNA damage (Comet assay is an example).**

- **Gene expression (Oncogenes, stress proteins).**

- **Altered enzyme activity (Radical pairs).**

- **Immune system perturbations.**

- **Endocrine disruption (Melatonin for example).**

- **Altered blood-brain barrier.**

- **Autonomic nerve function (EEG, ECG).**

- **Sleep or circadian rhythm disruption.**

- **Headaches, neurological effects.**

- **Reproduction disorders.**

- **Carcinogenesis (Brain, leukemia).**

EMI can be classed as narrow-band or wide-band:

Narrow-band EMI sources can be:

- Smart meters/smart devices/automatic meter readers (AMR)/advanced metering infrastructure (AMI) utility wireless networks.
- Two way radios (transceivers).
- Cordless phones, mobile phones and cell phones.
- Wireless scanners and wireless checkout devices.
- Radio frequency identification devices (RFID).
- Wi-Fi networking.
- Television and radio transmission towers.
- Cell phone towers.
- RADAR systems.
- Rural internet and satellite internet.

Here are some sources of wide-band EMI:

- Computers.
- Cathode ray tube (CRT) TV's.
- Digital flat screen TV's.
- Power lines.
- Electric switches and relays.
- Electric motors.
- Variable frequency drives (VFD).
- Thermostats.

- Bug zappers.

- Inverter systems.

- Florescent lights.

- Compact florescent lights (CFL).

- Light emitting diode (LED) lights.

- Neon signs.

- Stereo systems.

- MP3 players.

- Electronic lamp dimmers.

- Cars.

- Transportation systems.

- Electric and electronic toys.

- Battery powered watches.

- Cordless, cell and smart phones.

- Anti-static devices.

- Electrical grounding systems.

Basically, most digital equipment will have broadband emissions from it. If it is switching a large amount of power, then it may produce large amounts of electromagnetic interference.

The pictures on the following pages show the effects of electromagnetic interference on the human body voltage.

The Human Body Voltage

The human body voltage appears like a capacitor charging and discharging when in contact with conductive flooring that is electrically grounded.

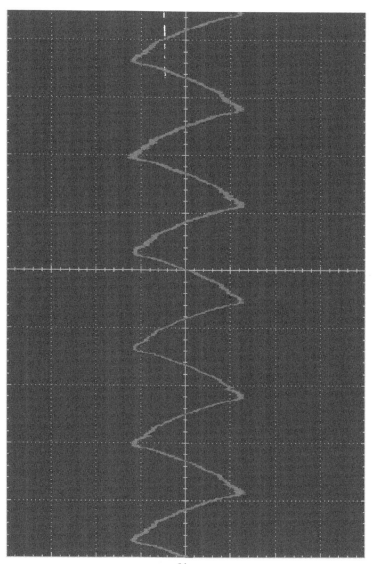

The Human Body Frequency Spectrum

A fast Fourier transform (FFT) reveals the many frequencies of electrical energy induced into the human body from contact with the conductive flooring.

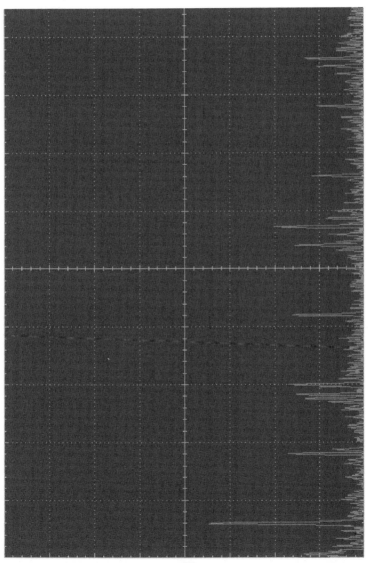

There was a shift that occurred largely in the 1980's from analogue electronics to digital electronics. Analogue electronics did not have a digital microprocessor chip in it and was made out of many basic electronic components. More importantly, it did not have the high speed pulsing that characterizes digital electronics. It is this high speed pulsing that causes digital electronics to be generally very dirty electromagnetic interference producing equipment.

Digital electronics uses electrical square waves to drive it. A square wave is one of the dirtiest electrical waves and as such it has many harmonics associated with it. Harmonics are the many different frequencies of waves that must be added together to produce the square wave. Basically, if you have a 60 Hertz square wave, then it will contain many higher frequencies of waves to produce it. They may be thousands of times higher in frequency than the wave that they are part of. It is for this reason that a standard AM radio when tuned into static can detect electrical noise. It is the harmonics that it is detecting in the square wave.

Computers function on high speed switching of square waves. For this reason you will find some very interesting microwave, radio, electric, and magnetic fields around them. The fields vary with the age of the computer and the different brands of computers. Laptop computers can be a particular problem due to the electronics being located below the keyboard and mouse pad. Some of these areas underneath can have very high levels of EMI producing electronics! It is best with a laptop computer to switch to a large font on the display, push the laptop back, and use a separate keyboard and mouse to control it.

When reviewing the BBC News article "*Scientists question if wi-fi laptops can damage sperm*", we find:

"Scientists are questioning if using wi-fi on a laptop to roam the internet could harm a man's fertility, after lab work suggested ejaculated sperm were significantly damaged after only four hours of exposure."

Florescent lights, compact florescent lights (CFL), and light emitting diode (LED) lights appear to produce radio waves from their power switching electronics. These radio emissions appear to vary between the different sizes of light bulbs and also how old they are. It is not a good idea to bring radio frequency producing equipment into your environment and for this reason I advise people against using these products. Testing has shown that these products can couple their electromagnetic fields into water and cause stray voltage effects. This is a concern due to the human body being 70% to 90% water, depending on age.

High electromagnetic interference lighting products are a serious issue when mounted to ceilings that are underneath an upper story. The fields that are coming out of them will make hot zones of electromagnetic radiation in the areas of the flooring above! They may also put harmonics on the electrical cables that run underneath the floor and create extensive electromagnetic interference fields wherever they run.

This is shown in the next picture.

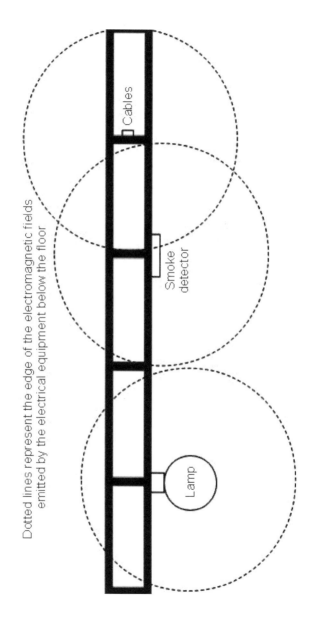

Under-Floor EMI

Electromagnetic fields come up through flooring from electrical products below

Dotted lines represent the edge of the electromagnetic fields emitted by the electrical equipment below the floor

Cables

Smoke detector

Lamp

Hairdressing products have some interesting electromagnetic fields around them and the hairdryer is perhaps one of the worst. The hairdryer consumes a large amount of current and has a brush motor inside it. Brush motors create sparks and this leads to wide band radio wave emissions near to it. It also puts dirty electricity into the electrical system. Hair clippers have large magnetic fields, corded ones put large AC voltages onto the human body, and the cordless ones appear to emit radio waves. It is concerning that these are used near to the head and it is probably a good idea not to expose developing children to these products.

Florescent tanning booths and beds may be an electromagnetic interference hot zone and should probably be avoided. The tanning light spectrum may be an issue as well. Dr. John Nash Ott found that there appears to be a biologically harmful field near the ends of florescent tubes where the cathodes are located. He believed it was a source of X-ray emissions. The florescent tube electronics also produce electromagnetic fields that may be extensive.

Some of the new digital televisions (TV) appear to be producing levels of electromagnetic interference that are affecting peoples health. I measured electromagnetic interference that was produced by my digital TV at a distance of fifty feet away from it! The electromagnetic interference that this particular 32" LCD flat screen TV was producing appeared to be an interference type of radiation. There were pockets of low and high interference AM radio frequencies throughout the home. I had noticed plant deformity and leaf tip problems in the plants in the room of the digital TV which appeared to be caused by the electromagnetic interference. The interesting thing about discontinuing the use of my digital TV was that plants started to grow in my garden that had appeared dormant for years! Plasma TV's appear to be the worst offenders of the new digital TV's with large electromagnetic interference fields around some of them.

Regarding human health, you should ensure that you stay out of the electromagnetic fields of televisions. A good rule of thumb is that the detectable electromagnetic field is generally three times larger in all directions than the screen size. These fields pass straight though walls and can be very high on the other side of the wall behind the television.

This can be a problem in hotels. The problem that I have with the hotel bed is that literally inches from your head on the other side of the wall may be a very large flat screen TV that is radiating very large electromagnetic radiation fields! The rooms also appear to have energy star lighting products that create a variety of emissions in the room and the light may cause insomnia. When in a hotel, it makes sense to sleep with your head in the center of the room and not against the wall in order to ensure that your brain is not in any strange fields that may be coming through the wall.

You will find emissions of wide band radio waves, X-rays, electrostatic, electric, and magnetic fields around cathode ray tube televisions. In an effort to prevent X-ray emissions, the screen is impregnated with lead. As such, they are an excellent device to study the biological effects of electromagnetic radiation. I call them "the power line within your home" as they emit more powerful fields into the human environment than most utility power lines!

It is quite possible that some of the illness and disease in the population are following the increase in television screen sizes!

Video games have brought children very close to the television. This means that their eyes are absorbing more of the artificial light and they may be spending extended time in the unnatural electromagnetic fields that the television produces. An interesting observation of autistic children is that it occurs 5 times more in boys than girls. Boys do tend to play more on video game systems than girls, and this may be a factor. The testicles are vulnerable to radiation exposures due to being external to the body.

Remote controls may be an issue, as they emit wide band radio wave emissions every time you use them! The transition from infrared to wireless radio frequency controllers is concerning and seems to be happening without any regard to the health symptoms that are being widely reported around wireless transmitting systems. Many video game systems now use transmitting wireless controllers and they may be able to affect the health of developing children and adults.

Solar photovoltaic (PV) power systems on the roofs of residential homes may be an issue. The inverter system that converts the direct current electricity from them into alternating current appears to cause electromagnetic fields to occur on the equipment. The large scale adoption of solar photovoltaic systems in the home has not yet been around long enough to fully understand the health risks that they may present.

Electronic inverter system exposure is shown on the following pages. The higher the power of the system, the larger the electromagnetic interference from them may be.

Inverter Systems and Human Health

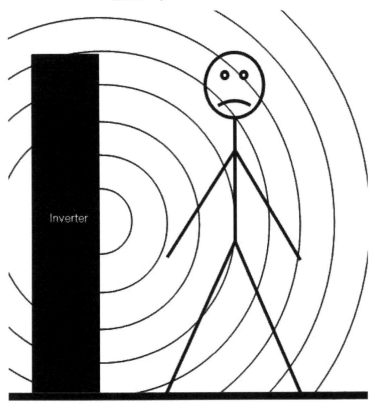

Many inverter systems create electromagnetic fields around
them. You should be wary about ontoring these fields.
Extended exposure to inverter systems may be harmful to
human health.

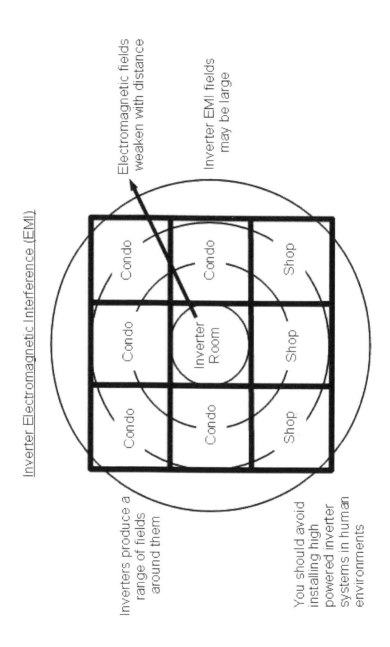

Inverter Electromagnetic Interference (EMI)

Electromagnetic fields weaken with distance

Inverter EMI fields may be large

Condo

Condo

Shop

Condo

Inverter Room

Shop

Condo

Condo

Shop

Inverters produce a range of fields around them

You should avoid installing high powered inverter systems in human environments

Due to the advent of digital equipment, the electrical circuits of the home may need to have line terminators installed in them. Line terminators prevent digital reflections from occurring on the home wiring. Essentially, it is an electrical noise reduction technique that can be used to reduce the home wiring electromagnetic interference emissions.

The radial electrical circuit is shown on the next page. The last socket may now need a line terminator installing into it to terminate the circuit to prevent electronic noise reflections from occurring. A line terminator is generally a small capacitor in parallel with a high impedance bleed resistor. This would be connected across the live and neutral terminals of the final socket in the radial circuit.

Terminating Radial Circuits

Radial electrical circuits may need line terminators installing at the last outlet.

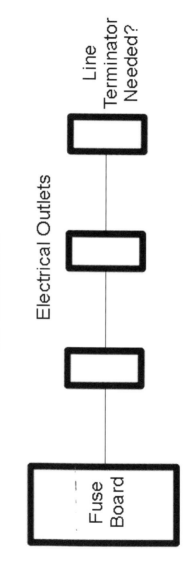

Electrical Outlets

Line Terminator Needed?

Fuse Board

Line terminators prevent frequency reflections from occurring on the circuit. A line terminator is generally a capacitor and a resistor.

Cars and transportation systems can have high amounts of EMI associated with them. In the past this came from their ignition systems and could be heard on the car radio as a buzzing sound that would increase in line with the revolutions per minute (RPM) of the car engine. Today, there is likely to be more electromagnetic interference from the electronic systems of the car and this may include:

- Radio frequency identification devices (RFID).
- Hybrid drive system.
- Electric drive system.
- Engine computer system.
- Global Positioning Systems (GPS).
- Alternating current (AC) inverter system.
- Entertainment systems.
- Cell phone charger.
- Cell phone.

People who have traced their sickness to their cars often change to a basic model of diesel car. They report improved health due to the lack of an ignition system in the diesel engine. I had intense intestinal pains after working with a car ignition system. The risk appears to be greatest when working near to the battery, coil and spark plugs.

When characterizing electromagnetic radiation emissions from transportation systems, they should be measured at various speeds, and also during hard acceleration and hard braking. Dr. Samuel Milham reports that he discovered that the rotating wheels were producing significant magnetic fields in the human occupied areas of the cars he tested at speed.

Using your cell phone in the car is a bad idea due to the radio frequency reflections that may occur. This may raise the radiation environment in the car and may cause interference effects that may be harmful to human health. Not to mention the distraction effect that may lead to a collision!

Electromagnetic interference is occurring with motorbikes and appears to be much stronger due to the compactness of a motorbike. Many motorbikes have their battery and electronic systems mounted under the seat and this area may emit the most electromagnetic interference into the rider. More details on this can be found in the book "Motorcycle Cancer?" by Randall Dale Chipkar.

Electric bicycles are becoming popular and may have similar problems as motorbikes. The dynamo electric lighting system for bicycles may be an issue.

Entertainment systems in cars and planes are an interesting concept. Generally you will find the television mounted into the head rest. As such, there may be a large electromagnetic field around the headrest. Car sickness or jet lag? You may have been excessively exposed to electromagnetic radiation from the television system in the head rest!

The move to hybrid and electric cars appears to be taking place with little concern to the electromagnetic interference environment inside the car. There are reports of people detecting electromagnetic interference fields within these cars that can far exceed the 2 milli-gauss magnetic fields that the International Agency for Research on Cancer (IARC) have set as their limit for constant magnetic field level for safe human health. Other people have noticed that their children appear fatigued on a long drive in a hybrid car as opposed to a normal car. Hybrid cars and electric cars appear to emit high electromagnetic interference during acceleration that may be around 100 milli-gauss and up to 30 milli-gauss when cruising. Constant fields of 2 milli-gauss and above should be avoided due to the elevated cancer risk.

The Prius acceleration problems may have a link to electromagnetic interference in some cases. Strange electromagnetic fields can affect the human mind and cause confusion. People may think they are pressing the brake, when they are actually pressing the accelerator! I can recall times when I have been working around electronic equipment and have displayed this type of confused behavior. I have also seen people that I have supervised display it too! Generally, the people that you are with notice your error and correct you.

Cars may be filled various levels of electromagnetic radiation and interference fields that may make you sick. Before buying one of these, you should ask for the following information: Peak values of magnetic field, electrostatic field, electric field, and wide band radio field in the human occupied areas. You should also establish if the fields are pulsating.

It makes sense to be a late adopter of electric car technology. There may be many types of electromagnetic interference fields around them. It will be interesting to see if brings a wave of electromagnetic hypersensitivity (EHS) and disease into the lives of the owners. Riding around in an electric car may be comparable to sitting under utility power lines.

The home electric car charger may be an issue. It will draw a lot of current from the utility system and may cause dirty electricity effects to appear throughout your home. It may also raise the electromagnetic fields around the utility power lines in the area.

Your children may already be driving electric cars! Electric cars for children have been available for quite some time and there may be extensive electromagnetic fields around some of them. You are probably better off staying away from high powered electrical toys like this.

You should establish where the battery(s) is located. I have noticed that on buses that the seat that the driver sits in commonly has the batteries located underneath it! This is an undesirable configuration for human health and the battery(s) should be located with the engine, preferably as far away from the vehicle occupants as is possible.

Electrical, electronic and wireless toys are just a really bad idea around developing children. Some toys will have a wide range of electromagnetic fields around them. If you are going to have electrical toys around

**your children, you should assess the electromagnetic
interference that it produces before giving it to them.**

Electric toothbrushes can have high electromagnetic fields
around them and are used near to the brain, so you should
consider not using these around developing children.

**It is well known that frequent travelers have a high
obesity risk. Transportation systems of all types can
produce high electromagnetic interference
environments. Airplanes, buses, and trains may be
filled with electromagnetic interference and it is added
to by people using their electronic devices on them.**

The recent transition back to electric trams running through
the streets is an interesting concept. The overhead power
cable has current running through it that is returned through
the grounded rails in the road. This will set up
electromagnetic fields between them where the people are
riding. The harmonics on the current may set up radio
frequency emissions. If you ride daily on trams, you
should pay attention to your long term health and be aware
that you may develop electromagnetic hypersensitivity
conditions in the long term. Electric trains may have
similar issues. The EMI fields may extend along the route
of the tram, even when the tram is not in view. You should
avoid driving in the vicinity of electric tram tracks due to
the EMI emissions from them. The overhead cables and
tram tracks are shown in the next photograph.

Electric Trams and Trains

These may have a wide variety of electromagnetic interference emissions associated with them. An electromagnetic field may be set up in between the overhead power cables and the tram tracks below.

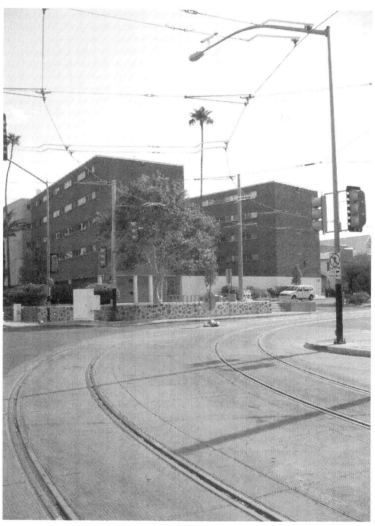

Airplanes have extensive electromagnetic emissions from their RADAR system and jet engines. The overhead cable that powers the tram may have dirty electricity emissions on it. The electric train may be emitting extensive EMI in some areas of it, especially near the electric motors and wheels. A ship will have RADAR and communications emissions.

Regarding airplanes, the pilots and air hostesses have high levels of sickness. The airplane has very high sources of electromagnetic radiation and these can be:

- High altitude solar radiation.
- Elevated cosmic radiation levels.
- Close proximity to lightning storms.
- RADAR.
- Communications systems.
- Engines.
- WiFi.
- Entertainment systems.
- Airplane control systems.
- Passenger electronics.
- Artificial lights.

The airport security area is a problem due to the scanners. Extended exposure to these systems has not been effectively studied and may be a long term health risk. It is not a good time to be a frequent air traveler.

Elevators may be an issue. Most elevators are essentially large Faraday cages that go whizzing up and down metal filled elevator shafts. You may find strange electromagnetic fields around elevators. These are added to by the electrical and electronic products within the elevators. Elevators typically have motors, florescent lights and control electronics within them. Regarding the lights, they are generally closer to your head due to the lower ceiling height and the electromagnetic fields will be stronger. You should avoid renting the apartment next to the elevator shaft due to the EMI effects. It is also preferable to use the stairs.

High voltage electric security fences are known for their high levels of EMI. These have similar problems to power lines and earthing and we will look into these problems later in the book. The electronics that power the security fence may have high EMI emissions from them and you should locate the electronic controller far from the human environment. These electric fences are usually found in farms and on top of high security walls.

Electronic lamp dimmers are one of the biggest culprits for producing electromagnetic interference effects within the home. I was quite surprised to find that a large and extensive electromagnetic field that I was detecting throughout a home was coming from a lamp dimmer! Lamp dimmers can completely fill a home with electromagnetic interference. You should avoid these products and instead use the three way filament lights instead.

Lamp dimmer effects are shown in the following pictures.

Lamp dimmers can create a very distorted current waveform.

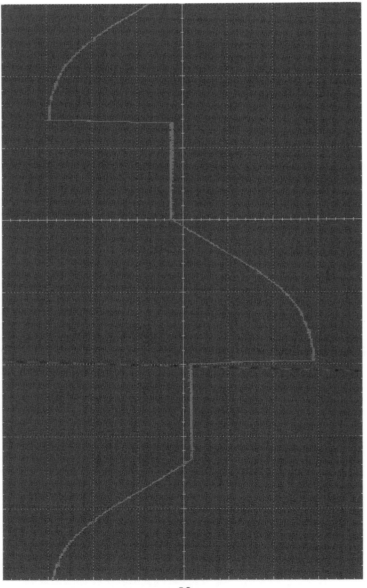

Lamp dimmers put a wide range of frequencies onto the electrical system. These harmonic and electrical noise frequencies can create large fields around the cables that may completely fill the home.

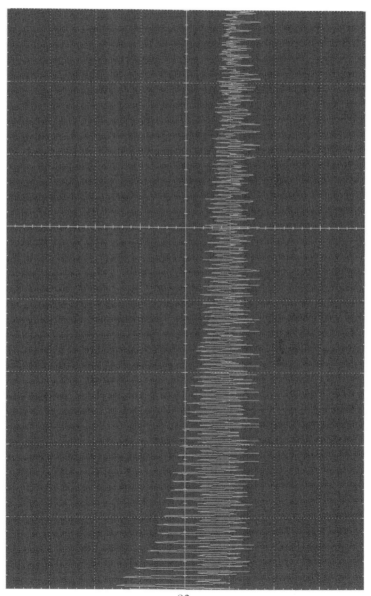

Microwave ovens can produce similar effects. I have detected extensive radio, microwave, and magnetic fields around these and, as such, I no longer use one. They make cell phones look safe!

People have started to realize that computer Wi-Fi networks, cell phone networks, DECT cordless phones, radio frequency identification (RFID) systems and the like are all causing biological problems. Wireless equipment should be avoided where possible. When using wireless equipment, the wireless transmission energy density is at a maximum next to the equipment and fades with distance. You should not place the transmitting equipment next to people or developing children. It is suggested that the wireless router be placed at least twenty feet from where people spend time. RFID security door systems should be avoided and it is preferable to use a standard key.

You are probably inadvertently spending time in these electromagnetic interference fields and do not realize it. The next diagram shows how this may be occurring in your environment.

Home Electromagnetics

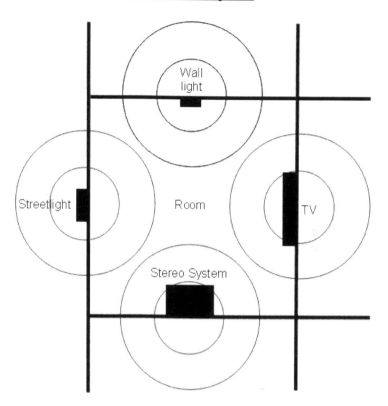

Electromagnetic field size will be dependent on each product
and some will be larger than others

When reviewing the Popular Science article *"The Man Who Was Allergic to Radio Waves"* we find that Per Segerback *"noticed his first symptoms -- dizziness, nausea, headaches, burning sensations and red blotches on his skin -- in the late 1980s, a decade into his telecommunications research work. All but two of the 20 or so other members of his group reported similar symptoms, he says, although his were by far the most severe. His EHS worsened and now, he says, even radar from low-flying aircraft can set it off."*

Electromagnetic hypersensitivity (EHS) has been extensively documented in plants and trees around these electromagnetic fields. The biological effect in plants and trees is not new, it was extensively researched and documented by Dr. John Nash Ott in the 1950's. Indeed, I have grown plants in electromagnetic fields that exhibited the growth defects that he documented.

This is shown in the next photograph. The three plants all looked the same when I bought them. They are all Dieffenbachia's and they all looked like the bushy one on the left. The center plant changed its growth in a Wi-Fi and AC electric field location. The right plant changed its growth in a wide band radio wave field that was produced by a 32" LCD digital television and now has very small and glossy green leaves with no patterning, as shown in the following picture. As you can see, they look like completely different species of plants and I call them my "Frankenstein" plants!

Exposure to EMI can cause plant deformity and growth defects. The leafy plant on the left is how the spindly ones to the right used to look before EMI exposure. You can see that there are significant problems with leaf growth, leaf patterning, and stem branching.

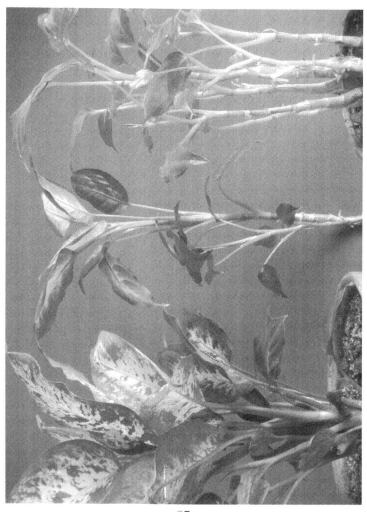

On the left is a normal fully grown Dieffenbachia leaf. On the right is a fully grown Dieffenbachia leaf from the plant in the EMI field produced by my 32" LCD TV. As you can see, their leaf growth and patterning is quite different!

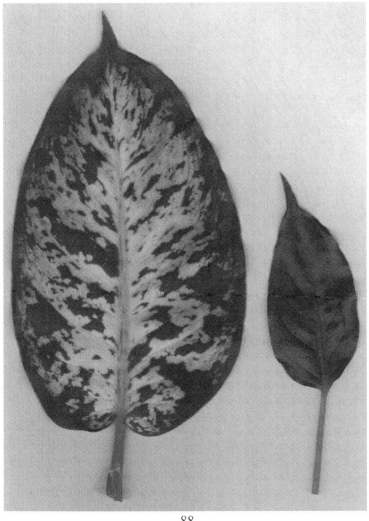

This Dieffenbachia plant was grown in a modern office environment that has wireless networking, computers, electronic florescent lighting products, and air conditioning. The leaf growth is very small and it appears to be a stunted version of the original plant.

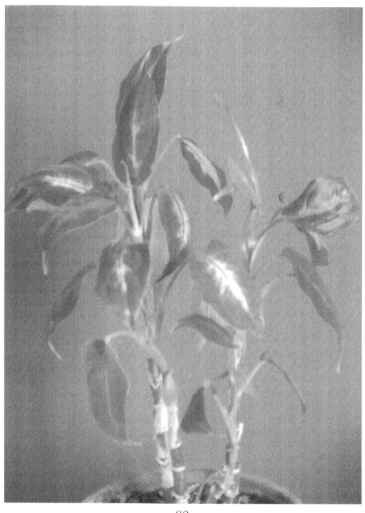

Babies and children are the most sensitive to the effects of EMI and particular attention should be paid to their environments. In a home with children you should avoid:

- Ionizing smoke detectors.

- Wireless baby monitors.

- Electrical toys.

- Electronic toys.

- Radio controlled and wireless toys.

- Train sets and car race tracks that may produce sparks.

- Battery operated wristwatches.

- Avoid placing the baby to sleep on a party wall with your neighbor as you will not know what EMI producing equipment is on the other side of that wall.

- Avoid placing the baby to sleep near an electrical outlet.

- Avoid having electrical cables running along the floor where the baby may crawl.

- Avoid letting a baby crawl on a floor that may have electrical cables running underneath it. (Upper story of a home).

- Avoid living in apartments, as these present the biggest electromagnetic interference risk from the neighbors around you. A detached house is far better.

- Avoid letting a baby crawl on any type of electrically conductive flooring, such as tile or concrete.

- Keep babies and children away from electrical, electronic and wireless equipment in general.

The next diagram shows some of these concepts with regards to furniture layout. Note that the wall light has been removed in the "good" picture. The streetlight is still shown, as you may not have any control over that. The sofa's are no longer against the walls to move them out of the fields of the electrical cables and any electrical equipment that may be on the other side of the wall. The bed has been moved out of the TV fields.

Electromagnetic Room Layout

Bad

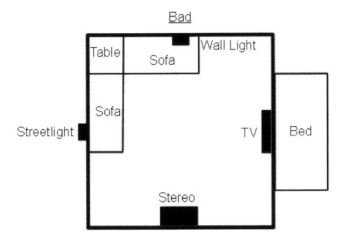

Good

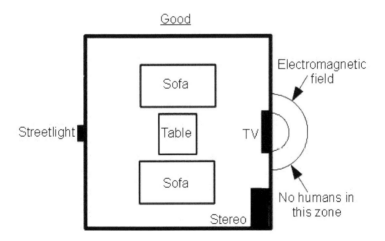

Women may be particularly at risk from the effects of electromagnetic interference exposures from electrical products. They generally wear under wired bra's and metal jewelery. These may couple into the fields through a process known as "induction" and AC voltages and frequencies will appear between the various items of metal on the body. It is easily measured using a digital multimeter or an oscilloscope with a frequency analyzer.

Measuring the AC voltage and frequency of the under wired bra is shown on the next page.

Electromagnetic Under Wired Bra

Metal under wired bra's have AC voltages and frequencies on them when in electromagnetic fields

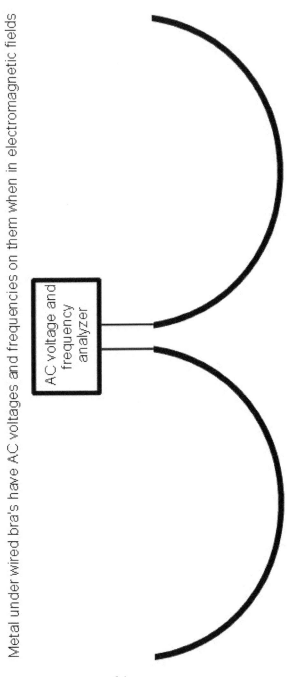

AC voltage and frequency analyzer

Students are a particularly high risk group, as they tend to live in very small rooms equipped with a microwave oven, refrigerator, television, computer system, cell phone and Wi-Fi. The most concerning product is the refrigerator, as it runs almost continuously. While the motor is running, it will be emitting a large electromagnetic interference field. Students should not sit or sleep next to refrigerators!

Students should also be aware of the products their neighbors have and where they are located on the other side of the wall. They should ensure that there are no electromagnetic interference producing items near to the walls of their beds and their desks.

It is preferable not to have any AC cables near to the bed and to pull the bed out from the wall to move it away from the fields of the electrical cables in the wall. The optimum position for your head is the center of the room when in bed. This will ensure that the field strength is at its lowest for the brain.

If the student room is equipped with a florescent light, then do not use it. Instead, use filament lighting products with stand lamps and desk lamps. If it has a window mounted air conditioner, stay at least ten feet away from it when in use.

Shift workers are a group of people who are much sicker than the general population. Extended exposure to artificial lighting, dirty electricity, radio and microwave transmitters, and computer screens are environmental factors that may be feeding into their illness. Unnaturally overriding the natural wake and sleep cycles of the human body does not help either.

"There are many examples of the failure to use the precautionary principle in the past, which have resulted in serious and often irreversible damage to health and environments. Appropriate, precautionary and proportionate actions taken now to avoid plausible and potentially serious threats to health from EMF are likely to be seen as prudent and wise from future perspectives."

Professor Jacqueline McGlade

Ionizing Radiation

Wikipedia states:

Ionizing (or ionising) radiation is radiation composed of particles that individually can liberate an electron from an atom or molecule, producing ions, which are atoms or molecules with a net electric charge. These tend to be especially chemically reactive, and the reactivity produces the high biological damage caused per unit of energy of ionizing radiation.

Natural background radiation comes from five primary sources: cosmic radiation, solar radiation, external terrestrial sources, radiation in the human body and radon.

Exposure to ionizing radiation causes damage to living tissue, and can result in mutation, radiation sickness, cancer, and death.

Ionizing radiation is commonly found in smoke detectors through their use of americium. Americium is commonly sourced from reprocessed nuclear fuel out of nuclear reactors. It is radioactive for hundreds of years and is used to ionize the air that passes through the detector to enable the detection of smoke particles.

Ionizing smoke detectors unnaturally raise the background radiation levels in the human environment.

The interesting thing about ionizing smoke detectors is that they are not needed. Photocell smoke detectors have always been available that do not use a radiation source to detect the smoke. After I realized that I had six ionizing smoke detectors installed at my home, I changed them out for photocell detectors instead. You will see them commonly marketed as kitchen smoke detectors, as they are not as sensitive as the ionizing type.

Fall out radiation is also ionizing and the world started to get coated in nuclear fallout radiation from the 1940's onward. Fall out radiation occurs when nuclear bombs are exploded and when nuclear power plants lose control and meltdown. Fallout radiation is spread around the world through the weather systems and as such, there is no place on the surface of the Earth that has not been contaminated. The effects of fallout radiation started to be realized in the 1960's and the nuclear weapons tests were moved underground in an effort to prevent this. Unfortunately, the nuclear surface contamination of the Earth will be emitting ionizing radiation for a few thousand years to come.

It is interesting to note that the USA government has stayed quiet on the issue of radiation fallout over the USA from the Fukushima nuclear power plant disaster in March 2011. The USA has constructed the largest radiation monitoring system in the world and will know exactly how much and where radiation was dropped onto the USA from that accident. Universities and independent researchers have been publishing data and it appears that the fallout was extensive and continuing daily as the Japanese nuclear power plant continues the process of melting down.

When reviewing the Los Angeles Times article
"Radioactive particles from Japan detected in California kelp", we find:

"Radioactive particles released in the nuclear reactor meltdown in Fukushima, Japan, following the March 2011 earthquake and tsunami were detected in giant kelp along the California coast, according to a recently published study."

The Fukushima disaster is going to be remembered by future historians as where humanity gained its knowledge of the effects of widespread nuclear contamination of the ocean, of Japanese nuclear power plant workers and the surrounding population.

Cathode ray tube televisions and florescent tubes may emit X-rays and this is ionizing radiation. For this reason, your cathode ray tube television has lead impregnated into the screen in an effort to prevent this.

The medical and dental field has been routinely performing X-rays of patients for many decades now and this is a source of ionizing radiation for the human mind and body.

Regarding X-Ray machines, occasionally one will be melted down during the recycling of metal and will contaminate the entire batch of metal with ionizing radiation! Some of this radioactive metal does make it back into the marketplace and many people unknowingly have it in their homes. It may even be in your metal coil mattress! It is a good reason to own a Geiger counter so that you can detect these radioactive contaminated metals.

A side effect of ionizing radiation is that it extends the human life span by stressing the body. It is quite possible that exposure to ionizing radiation sources has increased the human life span from an average age of 65 in the 1940's to an average age of 78 today. Age extension by ionizing radiation is extensively documented in the nuclear industry.

The problem of increasing the human life span from 65 to 78 is that there may be 20% more people on the planet than really should naturally be here. With a world population of 7 billion, it is possible that 1.17 billion of them should not be here! This increasing population is raising pollution levels and stressing the world food supplies.

You will also notice it in Japan. Japan had two nuclear bombs dropped on it in 1945. This coated Japan with extensive fallout radiation that raised the background radiation levels. The people of Japan are noted for their longevity. It is quite possible that these longed lived people had just the right amount of radiation exposure from the natural sources and the fallout during their lives to reach the peak of longevity. Unfortunately, too much ionizing radiation will shorten the human lifespan by inducing disease into the body.

Stressing the human body with ionizing radiation is called "Radiation Hormesis". Wikipedia states:

Other analyses have shown persistent depression of peripheral leucocytes and neutrophils, increased eosinophils, altered distributions of lymphocyte subpopulations, increased frequencies of lens opacities, delays in physical development among exposed children, increased risk of thyroid abnormalities, and late consequences in hematopoietic adaptation in children.

Ionizing radiation exposure is a complex equation and the correct radiation exposure for the human is always found in green environments with tree canopies.

The natural lifespan of humans in green environments is likely to be much shorter due to not having the cellular stresses of ionizing radiation exposure during their lives. Their bodies will live a shorter and healthier lifespan with excellent mental health before dying of natural causes. The correct human lifespan may be as short as fifty years of age away from radiation exposures.

Regarding the energy industry, Wikipedia states:

Nuclear reactors produce large quantities of ionizing radiation as a byproduct of fission during operation. In addition, they produce highly radioactive nuclear waste, which will emit ionizing radiation for thousands of years for some of the fission byproducts. The safe disposal of this waste in a way that protects future generations from radiation exposure is currently imperfect and remains a highly controversial issue.

Radiation emissions from high level nuclear waste decrease extremely slowly, which requires long term containment and storage for thousands of years before it is considered safe. During normal conditions, radioactive emissions from nuclear power plants are generally lower than coal-burning plants; though several high profile nuclear accidents have released dangerous levels of radioactivity.

There are a number of high radiation exposure occupations and Wikipedia lists them as:

- *Airline crew (the most exposed population).*
- *Industrial radiography.*
- *Medical radiology and nuclear medicine.*
- *Uranium mining.*
- *Nuclear power plant and nuclear fuel reprocessing plant workers.*
- *Research laboratories (government, university and private).*

Solar radiation is a source of ionizing radiation and many health symptoms have been linked to it. Indeed, it is well known that when solar flares erupt, that human health is affected. In particular, disease, suicide, war, aggression and famine has been linked to it. Sunspots can have a similar effect.

When reviewing the amateur-radio-wiki.net article *"Sunspot Cycle"*, we find:

"Most shortwave radio users know that there is a correlation between sunspots and propagation conditions. Sunspots are dark regions on the surface of the Sun, which are cooler than surrounding areas. They occur when the lines of the Sun's magnetic field become twisted. There are more sunspots when the Sun is more active, and produces more radiation which can affect the Earth's ionosphere."

From my experiments, it is clear that various radiation exposures have a poisoning effect on the human mind and body and stress it. It appears that the longer and sicker lifespan has replaced the shorter and healthier natural lifespan for many people.

We can get an estimation of how radiation affects cellular development by growing plants near sources of ionizing radiation. I am currently growing Dieffenbachia's (Dumb Cane) in the ionizing radiation fields of americium smoke detectors to see how this radiation will affect them.

Wikipedia states:

Americium is the only synthetic element to have found its way into the household...Americium is not synthesized directly from uranium – the most common reactor material – but from the plutonium isotope... Most americium is produced by bombarding uranium or plutonium with alpha particles in nuclear reactors – one tonne of spent nuclear fuel contains about 100 grams of americium.

The following pages show photographs of the experiments that I am currently performing using americium ionizing smoke detectors and plants.

A single ionizing americium smoke detector was used here. This is typical of what a home would have installed in the 1980's.

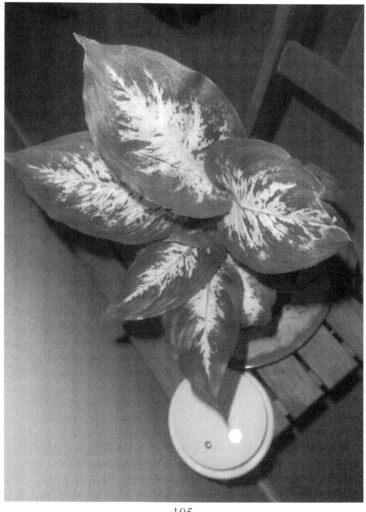

I found that my home had been constructed in 2004 with six ionizing americium smoke detectors and they were used to perform this experiment.

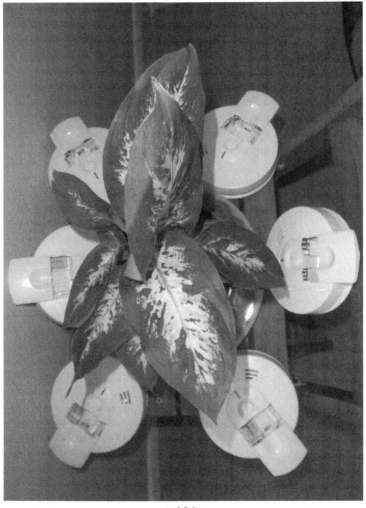

As can be seen, all of the plants died that were involved in this experiment. The control plant was inadvertently exposed to the radioactive ionizing americium smoke detectors during setting up the experiment and followed the same death process. It appears to be a case of "Delayed Radiation Complications".

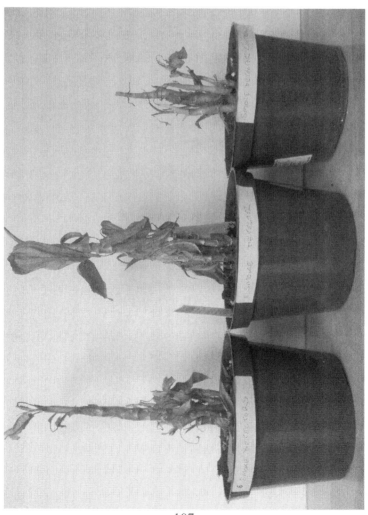

I ran the experiment again with cactus, due to cactus being a high radiation plant. I made sure that each cactus was not exposed to the radiation from the other cactus experiment.

I found that the six made in Mexico in 2004 smoke detectors did not harm the cactus but the one made in China in 2010 was particularly biologically harmful. The compliance monitoring group for the University of Arizona tested the two types of smoke detectors used with calibrated professional equipment. China detector figure first and Mexico detector figure is in brackets:

- Victoreen 451B ion chamber: 10-40 microrad per hour for both.
- Ludlum 44-9: 250(60)CPM
- Ludlum 44-3: 10,000(1,500)CPM.

Thank you to the University of Arizona for assisting in this experiment. As you can see, different types of americium smoke detectors can have greatly varying radiation readings. Since there is so much variability with residential americium smoke detectors, it is better not to use them and to use photocell smoke detectors instead. These are commonly sold as kitchen smoke detectors. The radiation stressed cactus is shown in the next photograph.

"My main frustration is the fear of cancer from low dose radiation, even by radiologists."

John Cameron

The single made in China smoke detector cactus was showing stresses that neither the control nor the cactus with six made in Mexico smoke detectors were showing.

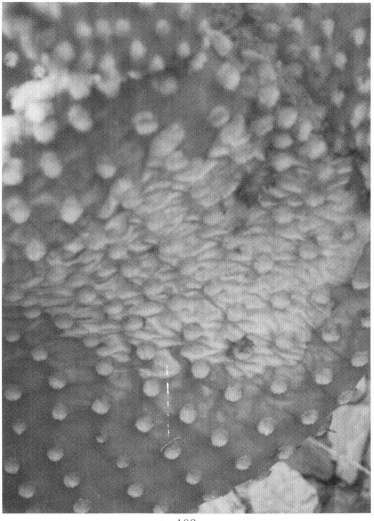

Wireless Radiation

Traditionally, the antenna has been a long piece of straight metal that is energized by electrical energy to electrify the surrounding environment. The length of the metal antenna is matched to the frequency of energy that it transmits. The receiving antenna is matched in length and will absorb that frequency of energy from the environment. The electricity that is absorbed by the receiving antenna is then amplified and turned into a useful signal by the system that uses it.

Antenna systems come in many forms and are commonly disguised. The toxicity of antenna systems has long been known. Indeed, the microwave oven was born out of RADAR system development. RADAR was known to heat the engineers who were working with the systems. The engineers who worked with RADAR knew that they could rapidly warm their lunches with the high powered systems!

The microwave oven is the highest power transmitting device in the home. Nothing else comes close to it. Several hundred watts of microwave energy that heats your food by vibrating the water molecules. For the longest time they were banned in Russia as their scientist had deemed the food unfit for human consumption. That is also my assessment of the situation.

If you measure the magnetic, wide band radio wave, and microwave fields around a microwave oven when it is in use, you will find extensive fields in the human environment that extend several feet out from it. These fields are patchy and may pulsate. Most electromagnetic radiation researchers believe the pulsating fields to be the most harmful to human health.

I no longer use my microwave oven. It is a health choice that I made based on research that I conducted on plants in electromagnetic fields. If an electromagnetic field can change the growth patterns in plants, then it probably has the ability to affect human cellular development. You can check to see if your microwave oven is leaking radiation by placing a cell phone inside it and calling it from another phone. If it rings, then your microwave oven is leaking radiation!

The microwave oven is the highest power antenna system in a home, but what is the next highest? It is your cellphone! Many cellphones have the ability to generate approximately 2 watts of transmission energy and they do it right next to your brain! Smart phones can have multiple transmitter systems in them that operate at different frequencies.

When reviewing the Scientific American article "*Mind Control by Cell Phone*",we find:

"The significance of the research," he explained, is that although the cell phone power is low, "electromagnetic radiation can nevertheless have an effect on mental behavior when transmitting at the proper frequency."

The interesting thing about this study is that it is talking about exposure to a single cell phone. If you work in a cubicle office with one hundred other people with cell phones and WiFi computers, what would the effect be?

The potential power levels would be 100 times 2 watt cell phones plus 100 times 0.1 watt WiFi. This comes out to 210 watts of radiation emissions!

It is well known that certain plants will deform next to cell phones. When reviewing the emfnews.org article *"Electromagnetic effects on Plant Seeds, Beans and Yeast"*, we find:

"Samples of plant seeds, beans, and yeast microorganisms were located in the close proximity to cellular phones. Cellular phones were operating in stand by mode during this experiment; in other words, experiment provided effects of the 'near' field. The significant difference was observed in the growth cycle of green beans, black beans and black seeds on the twelfth day."

You should avoid carrying your cellphone in your shirt pocket, as you will be placing the fields of it very close to your heart and lungs. It is a really bad idea to irradiate your organs with radio frequency radiation! You should carry it in a bag to keep it away from your body when not in use. Use the speaker phone feature to keep it away from your head when using it. Avoid the wireless headsets, as they will be irradiating your brain. Even when in standby, cell phones are communicating with the cell phone tower approximately every ten minutes.

It has taken many years and cellphones are now listed as possible carcinogens and it is likely only a matter of time before they become listed as carcinogenic. Smart people pay attention to "possibly carcinogenic" products and avoid them. After conducting my research on cellphones, I canceled my contract and then watched for withdrawal symptoms. These are the health effects that I saw in the weeks following turning off the cellphone in the order that they occurred:

- Aching bones: Right hand digits, left lower rib, left thigh bone and skull. This was in line with the locations where the phone would be carried or used.

- Fatigue.

- Three days after turning off the phone, I had two nights of insomnia.

- Tiredness in the morning that lasted approximately one month.

- Left thigh muscle was twitching and the nerves were tingling. This was the location where I would carry the phone.

- Rib cage pains.

- Approximately three weeks later, body and intestinal pains for 1 night only.

- Headache that lasted for two days.

- Strange dreams.

It appears that cellphones poison the mind and body with long term exposure. This poisoning effect has been observed in plants near to microwave transmitters and they show stunted and deformed growth patterns. To put this to the test, I devised an experiment to produce withdrawal symptoms in the human mind and body.

The test was very simple. I live very close to three cell phone towers. Each is between 2,000 feet and 2,300 feet from my home. I had identified mylar film as a radiation shielding product, as NASA uses it in spacesuits. Mylar film is commonly sold as thermal "Space" blankets for first aid kits. My experiment consisted of sleeping on top of three sheets of mylar film and under three more sheets of mylar film. I was shocked at how extensive the withdrawal was! Here is what happened:

- Night 1: Withdrawal started the very first night and comprised of general aches and pains. Poor sleep. Feeling of nausea. Low energy in the morning. Spent 8 hours in mylar film.

- Night 2: No aches and pains. Insomnia. Low energy in the morning. 8 hours spent in mylar film.

- Night 3: Mild pain in heart for a fraction of a second. Skull pains for a few hours. Mild insomnia with naps. Tired in the morning. Spent 8 hours in mylar film.

- Night 4: Mild insomnia with naps. Plenty of energy in the morning. Got up early. Spent 6 hours in mylar film. Spent 1 hour hiking outdoors in sunlight to help with the withdrawal.

- Night 5: Slept well. Minor aches and pains. 8 hours under mylar film.

- Night 6: Slept well. Minor pains in intestines and testicles. 8 hours under mylar film.

As you can see, it was an extensive range of symptoms that showed up. I was going to continue for longer, but the Sun had a solar flare, so I stopped the test. I stopped sleeping with the three sheets on top of me but continued to sleep with 3 sheets of mylar film underneath me. I didn't feel quite right, with headaches and fatigue. So after a couple of weeks I took the mylar film off the bed completely and this rectified the situation. I suspect that the mylar film was causing my body to be cycled between low and high radio frequency radiation levels daily and that was causing the problem. I later tested mylar film and found that it acts as an antenna system! So it appears that I was subjected to electromagnetic shielding that had radio frequencies on it.

After seeing this effect, I concluded that the only true solution to eliminate human man-made radiation exposure is to turn off the transmitters that are producing it. It is not realistic nor humane to expect people to move out of the area nor to electromagnetically shield their homes.

The computer WiFi units appear to be the next largest source. They are particularly concerning due to the fact that they are always broadcasting their signals into the human environment. They never switch off. The power level is low at 0.1 watt, but the continual exposure to a digital microwave signal is a bad idea. I no longer use WiFi at home for that reason. When siting your WiFi system, you should consider mounting the unit as far away from the human environment as possible. Distance helps lower the signal strength from the base unit. Many electromagnetic researchers call WiFi "*the cell phone tower within your home*" as higher wireless radiation power levels can be found near to them than what you can find around cell phone towers.

Cordless phones, cordless baby monitors, cordless video systems, cordless alarm systems and cordless weather systems should all be avoided. You should be aiming to keep your environmental electromagnetic radiation levels as natural as possible.

You should avoid transmitting systems in homes that have metal roofs, metal wall studs, metal in their walls (stucco), and metal siding. Metal does the following things in transmission fields:

- Reflects waves.
- Creates interference.
- Absorbs radiation.
- Re-radiates radiation.
- Focuses radiation which creates hot spots.

This is shown in the next diagram.

Metal Homes

EMI source

Metal homes may be filled with
electromagnetic radiation and interference,
and may be electrified

Structure
stray
voltage

The interesting thing about microwave radiation is that the atmosphere filters it out from the Space radiation. There were only extremely low levels of microwaves in the human environment until the human introduced high powered microwave transmission systems! For this reason you should be concerned. The use of microwaves for communications has raised the human microwave environment thousands of times higher than anything that can be found in nature! You have no genetic adaptation to high powered man-made microwave radiation.

You can replicate the atmospheric filtering effect with a cell phone. Simply put it in a see-through waterproof plastic bag and immerse it in water. About an inch into the water you will see the signal strength go to zero. This is because the water is absorbing the wireless radiation. The same process is occurring in your body when in wireless radiation fields. If there is a signal on your cell phone, then you are absorbing man-made wireless radiation. This may lead to your body becoming toxic and you will get a level of poisoning that could lead to electromagnetic hypersensitivity.

This is a concern with babies and developing children as their bodies are so much smaller. An inch of wireless radiation penetration into them is far deeper than on an adult! Wireless radiation will go very deep into a new born baby.

Regarding cell phone towers, they are generally regarded by electromagnetic researchers as being potentially toxic to the population who live within approximately a quarter of a mile of them. There are a number of studies that have shown that the illness rates spike up significantly in this quarter mile radius from the tower. The studies show that the illness rates are distance related. The closer you live to a cellular transmission tower, then the more likely it is that it will affect you.

Cell phone towers use the "sector antenna" that cover an area of 120 degrees. That is why you generally see a triangular arrangement of antenna systems to give the full 360 degrees coverage of the area. They typically cover a radius of 2 to 3 miles from the tower with good signal strength. This short transmission distance is the reason why you see cell phone towers at regular intervals in populated areas. Many cell phone towers are needed to give complete coverage in a city environment.

Homes near to transmitter systems may have radiation "hot spots" in them that extended time in these areas may lead to electromagnetic hypersensitiivty.

When reviewing the npr.org article *'Wi-Fi Refugees' Are Moving To West Virginia To Escape Radio Waves*, we find:

"Dozens of Americans who claim to have been made ill by Wi-Fi and mobile phones have flocked to the town of Green Bank, W.Va.," the BBC reports. They're heading there because of the area's "National Radio Quiet Zone" — 13,000 square miles that surround the National Radio Astronomy Observatory's Robert C. Byrd Green Bank Telescope. The zone, as Wired has reported, is "nearly free of electromagnetic pollution" because of regulations put in place decades ago. Those restrictions aim to keep other electromagnetic signals from interfering with the telescope's work.

People who live near cell phone towers should consider getting rid of their cell phones, Wi-Fi, and any wireless devices in the home. This action will reduce your radiation environment inside the home.

Directional antenna systems have what is known as "Side Lobe" emissions. The areas that the side lobes extend into are regarded as the most toxic areas for human health. They occur relatively close to the antenna system. Dish antennas are typical of this.

It is becoming common today for communication companies to disguise their antenna systems and you may not be aware of their presence. You should assume that there are transmission antenna systems in the following places:

- Police Stations.
- Fire stations.
- Hospitals.
- Military installations.
- Government buildings.
- Schools.
- Downtown areas.
- Television companies.
- Air and sea ports.
- Anywhere that you can get cellphone signals.
- Anywhere you can get WiFi signals.

- Anywhere that you can see communication towers.
- Anywhere where utility meters are present.

Firemen have gotten wise to the toxicity of cell phone towers and the International Association of Fire Fighters is opposed to them being located near to fire stations. This is their stance:

The International Association of Fire Fighters' position on locating cell towers commercial wireless infrastructure on fire department facilities, as adopted by its membership in August 2004, is that the IAFF oppose the use of fire stations as base stations for towers and/or antennas for the conduction of cell phone transmissions until a study with the highest scientific merit and integrity on health effects of exposure to low-intensity RF/MW radiation is conducted and it is proven that such sitings are not hazardous to the health of our members.

Further, the IAFF is investigating funding for a U.S. and Canadian study that would characterize exposures from RF/MW radiation in fire houses with and without cellular antennae, and examine the health status of the fire fighters as a function of their assignment in exposed or unexposed fire houses. Specifically, there is concern for the effects of radio frequency radiation on the central nervous system (CNS) and the immune system, as well as other metabolic effects observed in preliminary studies.

It is the belief of some international governments and regulatory bodies and of the wireless telecommunications industry that no consistent increases in health risk exist from exposure to RF/MW radiation unless the intensity of the radiation is sufficient to heat body tissue. However, it is important to note that these positions are based on non-continuous exposures to the general public to low intensity RF/MW radiation emitted from wireless telecommunications base stations. Furthermore, most studies that are the basis of this position are at least five years old and generally look at the safety of the phone itself. IAFF members are concerned about the effects of living directly under these antenna base stations for a considerable stationary period of time and on a daily basis. There are established biological effects from exposure to low-level RF/MW radiation. Such biological effects are recognized as markers of adverse health effects when they arise from exposure to toxic chemicals for example. The IAFF's efforts will attempt to establish whether there is a correlation between such biological effects and a health risk to fire fighters and emergency medical personnel due to the siting of cell phone antennas and base stations at fire stations and facilities where they work.

You can read the full article here:

http://www.iaff.org/hs/Facts/CellTowerFinal.asp

It is well known in the industry that extended exposure close to a transmitter system may be harmful to human health and you should always try to put distance between yourself and transmitting devices.

If you have a job that is located near to a high powered transmitter, then you should consider changing your job. Extended close exposure to a high powered

transmitter system should be expected to increase your chances of illness, disease, cancer and premature death.

Pay attention to your hearing, as you may develop "Microwave Auditory Effect". Wikipedia states:

The microwave auditory effect, also known as the microwave hearing effect or the Frey effect, consists of audible clicks (or, with modulation, whole words) induced by pulsed/modulated microwave frequencies. The clicks are generated directly inside the human head without the need of any receiving electronic device. The effect was first reported by persons working in the vicinity of RADAR transponders during World War II. These induced sounds are not audible to other people nearby. The microwave auditory effect was later discovered to be inducible with shorter-wavelength portions of the electromagnetic spectrum. During the Cold War era, the American neuroscientist Allan H. Frey studied this phenomenon and was the first to publish information on the nature of the microwave auditory effect.

If you start to hear strange things that no one else is, start looking into the transmitting devices around you!

The following pictures show building transmitters.

In this building and the surrounding buildings the people may be sick due to the transmissions from these multiple antenna systems. The worst place for human health may be the top floors of the building.

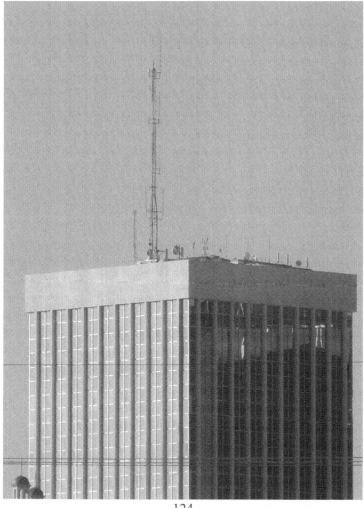

Transmitters on Buildings

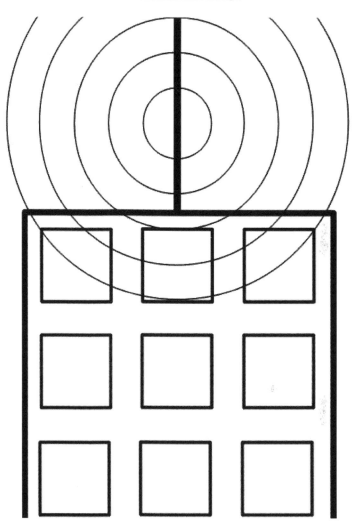

Can you see the cell phone antenna system?

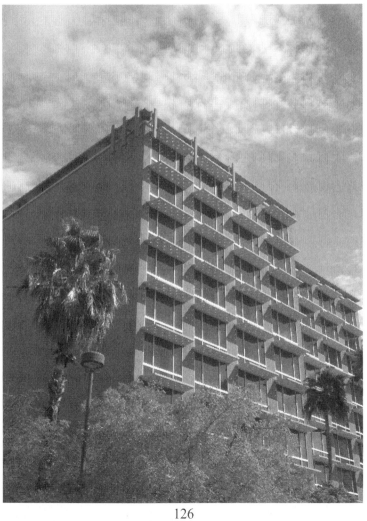

It is on the top corner of the building. One has to wonder how the people who stay in the hotel must feel? Tall hotels commonly have transmitter systems on their roofs and you should avoid staying in the upper floors.

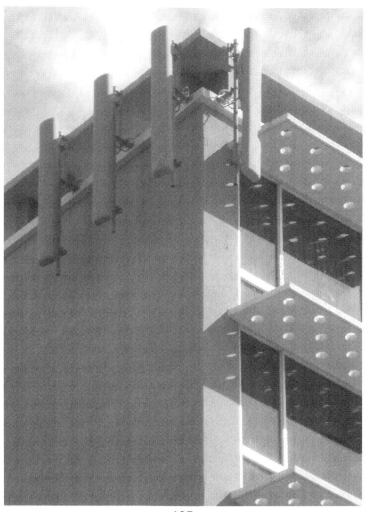

This cluster of radio frequency antennas, horns and dishes may be making the people in the area sick. Human habitations in the area of transmitting devices is a really bad idea.

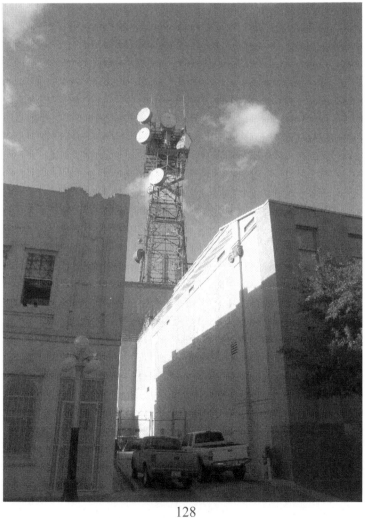

Police stations can have high powered transmitter systems and they may be a cause of "Angry Aggression Theory" as applied to police officers.

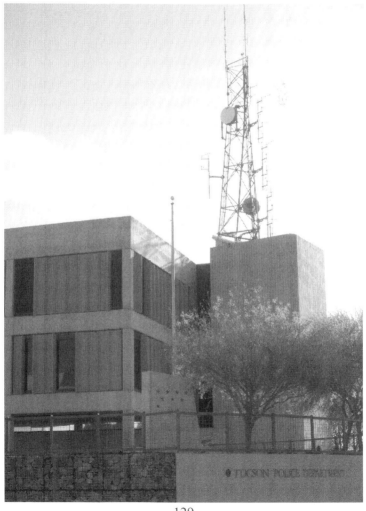

The military has developed antenna technologies for use against humans and they have known for a long time that they can make people sick with it and damage their long term health. These fall under the class of "electromagnetic weapons".

The utilities are installing wireless transmitting utility meters at homes in number of countries now, including the USA. A popular product that the utilities use is the Itron OpenWay wireless communications system which is installed throughout Tucson, Arizona. The manufacturer states:

The Itron OpenWay wireless communication equipment operates in the Industrial, Scientific and Medical (ISM) bands at frequencies from 902 MHz to 928 MHz and from 2,400 MHz to 2,483 MHz. Also, a small number of devices incorporate wireless modems operating at frequencies 824-849 MHz and 1,850-1,910 MHz designated for the cellular operators (Cell Relays constitute about 1% of all the OpenWay wireless devices and can be mounted on poles or as part of a meter).

Tucson utilities appear to be using 0.5 watt Itron 100G transmitting gas meters, 0.1 to 0.3 watt transmitting Itron Centron electric meters and 1 watt transmitting Itron 100W water meters. So each property can have up to 1.8 watts installed at them. The homes are close together in Tucson and in a home like mine where the neighbors utility equipment is near, you essentially can have up to 6 utility meters transmitting approximately 3.6 watts of energy at or very near to your property! Unfortunately some homes may have what is known as the "mesh node" or "repeater" transmitter which may be much higher powered and may transmit much more frequently. The utilities appear not to notify the home owners that have these "mesh node" and "repeater" transmitters at or near to their properties. Some utility meters have multiple transmitter systems in them, so you may get subjected to higher levels of radiation at multiple frequencies from them. The utilities are willfully making many people sick with their biologically toxic transmitting meters.

It has been known for many years that a subset of the population cannot tolerate the radiation emitted by transmitting utility meters and sickness results in these people. The utilities appear to be engaging in silence regarding this fact and they know that some of their customers develop electromagnetic hypersensitivity that is easily preventable but is commonly misdiagnosed as other conditions that may result in the person being placed onto prescription medication, losing their job, and possibly being placed onto disability. Their children may be the most affected and may not develop correctly.

It is important to note that many transmitters have a minimum distance that you should not get within, otherwise you will put yourself into known biological harm. The radiated transmitter power levels are much higher than stated closer to the transmitter and are of a "near field" exposure. For Itron Centron utility meters:

"RF Exposure (Intentional Radiators Only). In accordance with FCC requirements of human exposure to radiofrequency fields, the radiating element shall be installed such that a minimum separation distance of 20cm is maintained from the general population."

They also have co-location requirements that specifies a minimum separation distance from adjacent transmitting systems.

Wireless radiation is readily absorbed by the human. The human is 70% to 90% water and the radio waves that are in the environment react with water. In the communications industry this is called "Rain Fade". When it rains, the wireless radiation power levels reduce as the rain drops absorb the energy. The human body does the same thing!

When queried about how wireless radiation affects the human mind and body, the wireless radiation industry will commonly incorrectly state that the "skin effect" protects the human. The skin effect is an observation that high frequency currents will travel down the outside of a conductor and not the center of it. This effect was noticed during the development of high frequency electricity.

The human body is not a conductor, but rather a semiconductor. Different electrical process are taking place and it is clear today that the human mind and body can be greatly affected by these high frequency man-made exposures. The human skin evolved in a natural electromagnetic radiation environment and is now in a very unnatural man-made one that is making many people sick.

These harmful effects can be shown by growing plants in the electromagnetic fields. Dr. John Nash Ott extensively pioneered the field of electromagnetic radiation plant growth defects and his books on the subject are an interesting read. Like Dr. John Nash Ott, I have been able to deform plants with electromagnetic fields. This is what I have established:

- Found that Smart/AMR/AMI utility transmitting meters can have a toxic effect on the various biological systems that are near to them. The harmful biological effects can occur for at least 76 feet from some of the devices and can kill plants.

- Found that the radiation emissions from ionizing smoke detectors can retard cellular growth and may actually kill certain types of plants.

- Found that wireless radiation puts plants into a dormant state where they follow the changes in the seasons but do not actually grow nor bear fruits. They become sterile and stunted. Removing the wireless radiation exposures resurrects them.

- Found that wireless radiation affects the growth and branching structure of some plants. Plants that grow tall may instead grow low to the ground.

- Some vines will not grow into areas of biologically unnatural radiation.

- Found that wireless radiation fields are patchy and unpredictable. Just moving a few inches can be the difference between a plant being healthy or it being stunted and deformed.

- Found that pulsed radiation from wireless weather station sensors and wireless utility meters can really retard and deform plants that are close to them. In some cases they will kill the plants.

- Discovered that certain electromagnetic exposures deform and retard plant growth and when removed, the plant drops all of the previous deformed leaf growth and starts growing normal growth from the tips of electromagnetic exposed part of the plant. The previously exposed part of the plant stays bald.

- Discovered that certain plants in unnatural radiation fields will only grow leaves on their branch tips at the edge of the plant. The interior of the branches of the plant stay bald. This growth pattern rectifies itself when the unnatural radiation field is removed.

- Found that the pomegranate tree will drop all of its leaf growth when the harmful wireless radiation field is removed and put up new growth from its base. The existing branches stay bald. The following year, it will put new leaf growth on both the old and new branches and bear fruit.

- Found that certain plants in biologically unnatural electromagnetic fields will turn their normally patterned leaves into dark green glossy leaves with no patterning.

It appears that when analyzing wireless radiation exposures you should think of them as you would think of a Tesla coil. The Tesla coil was where wireless radiation devices were developed from. A Tesla coil can emit biologically harmful visible sparks over long distances, often exceeding 100 feet. Some electrical, electronic, and wireless devices appear to emit similar biologically harmful "invisible sparks" a comparable distance. I call this:

"The Tesla Coil Model of Biologically Harmful Invisible Electromagnetic Radiation"

The human mind and body cannot sense these biologically harmful invisible sparks and it slowly gets sick from exposure to them. The longer you are exposed to it, the more toxic you become. The range of these toxic electromagnetic fields varies with each device and is very unpredictable.

The leaf defects that the Dieffenbachia (Dumb Cane) plant displays in unnatural electromagnetic fields are shown in the following picture.

Leaf Deformities

The fully grown leaf deformities are shown. As you can see, a wide range of different size leaves can be generated, depending on the field type and strength that the Dieffenbachia (Dumb Cane) plant is exposed to.

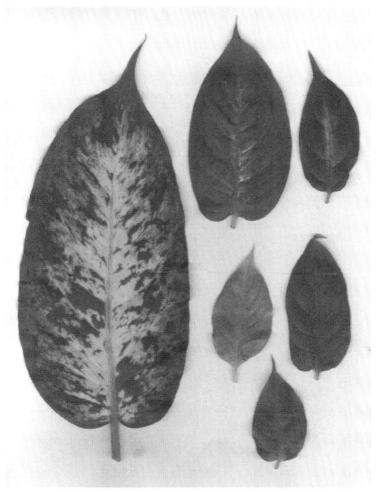

Regarding wireless transmitting devices, I have found after many plant growth experiments:

- Near exposures to transmitters are the most harmful. The most harmful transmitters that I have found are the lowest power ones that are sold to consumers as harmless wireless products! Devices that continually broadcast pulses of radiation every several seconds are the worst, such as wireless weather station sensors.

- Intermediate exposures are those from your neighbors wireless devices and those from Smart/AMR/AMI utility meters. These are the next worst exposures and you should be familiar with the wireless products that your neighbors have at their properties. You should consider installing electromagnetic shielding between the homes if they have harmful wireless products in use.

- Far exposures are those that are coming from high powered transmitters that are far away from your property. Examples of these are airport, port, and weather RADAR systems, TV and radio transmitters, government transmitters, cell phone towers, and so on. You should be aware of the locations of these to both your home and workplace. Only after working through the near and intermediate exposures should you start suspecting these as sources of your problems. Distance is your friend in the world of harmful electromagnetic radiation exposures!

My research is indicating that home wireless devices can produce a biologically toxic field close to them. The size of this harmful field varies from device to device. Some of the harmful fields from home devices can extend at least 76 feet and the field is very patchy. Some areas are fine and others are toxic. Regarding the toxicity of wireless radiation exposure from common devices in the home, a clear classification is now emerging about the level of toxicity of these devices.

The most biologically harmful fields appear to be produced by pulsed radiation devices that broadcast regularly. Smart/AMR/AMI utility meters and wireless outdoor temperature sensors are good examples. "Smart" enabled devices that are designed to integrate into your utility "Smart" meter are likely to behave in a similar fashion. Some Wi-Fi devices and smart phones also display this behavior and it may be related to the applications that they have installed on them. Automatic door opening RADAR sensors that are common in large stores may fall into this category.

After this, I have the Wi-Fi router exposure rated as the next most toxic device as it is broadcasting continuously in the home and workplace, make sure you do not sit near to them. You should use your computer on a wired network connection whenever possible and turn off the Wi-Fi. Some cordless home phones may be in this category as they appear to behave like wireless networks. Wireless game controllers and radio controlled toys are in this category.

The cell phone is in the third class of toxic devices and I recommend people to avoid them. They communicate with the cell phone tower every ten minutes or so. Each time they do so, they will fill your home with wireless radiation. If you have multiple phones in the home, then your home will be filled with wireless radiation every few minutes. Some types of cordless home phones may fall into this category.

The fourth class of wireless device appears to be devices that only broadcast a short wireless pulse when they sense an event that triggers them. A garage door open or closed sensor would fall into this category. Most wireless security sensors and wireless door chimes behave in the same way. Some wireless utility meters also can exhibit this behavior.

This is the classification that appears to be emerging for home wireless devices from most toxic to least toxic:

1. **Devices that emit regular pulses of wireless radiation at short intervals of every 60 seconds or less.**
2. **Devices that constantly emit wireless radiation.**
3. **Devices that emit pulses of wireless radiation every several minutes.**
4. **Devices that emit pulses of wireless radiation infrequently.**

If you have several wireless devices close together, then you may have to reassess which category they fall into as it will increase the frequency of wireless pulses and/or wireless energy power being transmitted.

The frequency that a wireless device operates on may increase the toxicity of it. The most toxic device I identified at my home was a wireless outdoor temperature and humidity sensor. It operates for about a year on two AA 1.5 volt batteries. The frequency that it operated at was 433.92 megahertz and it appeared to be deforming a wide range of plants for at least a 45 feet radius from the device.

The gas company later installed an Itron 100G gas meter that surpassed the biological toxicity of that device to the human. Installed 76 feet away from my bedroom, that device induced classic radio wave sickness into me! It is listed as operating at between 908 to 924 megahertz at up to half a watt of transmission power. Half a watt is high powered for a residential application that constantly transmits pulsed radiation every several seconds. It is unfortunate that the highest powered transmitting devices at your home may actually be the utility meters that you cannot switch off!

To sum up, the biological toxicity of a transmitter to a human depends on the following:

- Transmission power.
- Transmitting frequency.
- Modulation of the signal.
- Intermittent, pulsed or continuous transmission.
- Reflections and interference of the transmission.
- Distance from you.
- The fat to muscle ratio of your body.

- Metal implants.
- The amount of metal in your environment.
- The height above the ground that you live.

You should be very wary of where you keep your cellphone and men should avoid keeping it near to their testicles and women should avoid keeping it near to the breasts. You should avoid putting a cellphone in your shirt pocket as it will be irradiating your heart and lungs. You most certainly do not want to sleep with your cellphone under your pillow, but unfortunately, many children do this every night. It is preferable to carry a cellphone in a separate bag away from the body.

It is interesting to note that astronomers have always thought that a mass human radiation extinction would come from a solar flare or a supernova. Pulsars may present the biggest naturally occurring risk to human extinction, as they behave like pulsed wireless transmitters. As we know today, the pulsar radiation emission is far more harmful at much lower power levels than the continuous radiation emissions from the Sun or supernovas. This opens up the range of nearby astronomical objects that can threaten the Earth by orders of magnitude. As such, a human radiation extinction is far more likely to come from a pulsar than any other astronomical object!

When we talk about extinction, we must remember that this will also affect everything on the Earth. Human survival is completely dependent on plants. Plants are affected by many forms of radiation and I have performed numerous tests that show the biologically harmful effects from man-made radiation exposures.

Regarding the toxicity of wireless radiation exposures, this is the official stance currently:

Lyon, France, May 31, 2011: The WHO/International Agency for Research on Cancer (IARC) has classified radio frequency electromagnetic fields as possibly carcinogenic to humans (Group 2B), based on an increased risk for glioma, a malignant type of brain cancer, associated with wireless phone use.

I have found climbing vines will not grow into areas of harmful wireless radiation and that the Golden Pothos will lose the patterning on its leaves in these fields. This is shown in the following pictures.

Golden Pothos

The Golden Pothos will lose the patterning in its leaves when in harmful wireless radiation fields. They grow dark green.

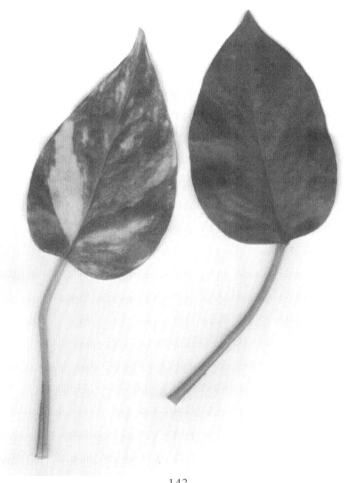

Climbing Vines

Some climbing vines will not grow into harmful wireless radiation areas. They provide an excellent indicator of the invisible patches of harmful wireless radiation that now exist.

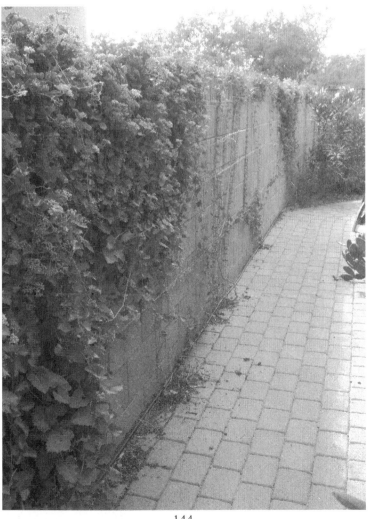

Electrical energy interacts with the natural fields of the Earth. The human is genetically adapted to interact with natural, weak magnetic and electromagnetic fields. The cities represent the opposite of what nature created and today are an alien environment for the modern human. As such, it is reasonable to say that the modern human is an alien having developed in such an alien environment.

The alien human is revealing itself in many ways. We can see it in the dramatic rise in childhood development problems. Autism, attention deficit disorder, hyperactivity, insomnia, depression, fatigue, and accelerated puberty are all problems that are prevalent in modern children. Autism is the most striking and has accelerated from being a rare problem in the 1970's where only 1 in 10,000 children were diagnosed with the condition to a common development issue where 1 in 40 boys have it today!

Autism has been following the rise in wireless communications for the last decade and this is shown in the next graph. The graph was complied from data presented by CTIA-The Wireless Association and Talk About Curing Autism (TACA). It is clearly an electromagnetic radiation disease. The longer the damaging effects of man-made electromagnetic radiation are denied, the more this graph will continue to increase. Unfortunately, the wireless radiation era is not a good time to be born into.

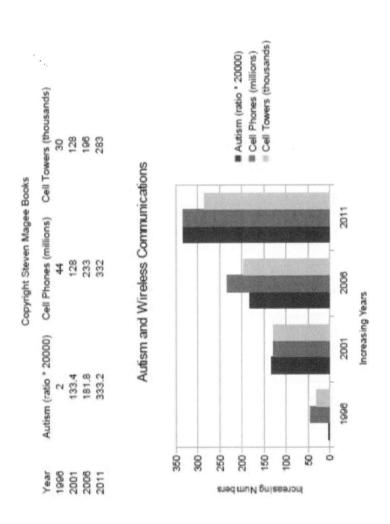

Copyright Steven Magee Books

Year	Autism (ratio * 20000)	Cell Phones (millions)	Cell Towers (thousands)
1996	2	44	30
2001	133.4	128	128
2006	181.8	233	196
2011	333.2	332	283

Autism and Wireless Communications

146

The BioInititaive 2012 report states:

The premise of this review is that although scant attention has been paid to possible links between electromagnetic fields and radiofrequency exposures (EMF/RFR) and Autism Spectrum Disorders (ASDs), such links probably exist. The rationale for this premise is that the physiological impacts of EMF/RFR and a host of increasingly well-documented pathophysiological phenomena in ASDs have remarkable similarities.

You can find out much information about transmitting systems by obtaining the FCC ID number. This is stamped on all transmitting systems and the presence of it reveals that the device has an intentional radiation transmitting device installed into it. This number can be typed into the FCC website at http://transition.fcc.gov/oet/ea/fccid/ to obtain many items that relate to it. You will commonly find the technical manual and the radio frequency data in amongst the FCC submittals by the manufacturer. It is a very useful resource for obtaining transmitter data. Press the "advanced search" button to be taken to a more advanced search menu with many more options on it.

If you find that you are being biologically damaged by a transmitter, then you can file a complaint to the FCC under rule 15. FCC rule 15 states that no transmitter may cause harmful interference. Simply state in your complaint that you have found harmful biological transmissions from an FCC approved device. List the health conditions and the FCC identification number of the device. Request the FCC to inform the operator of the FCC approved device to be notified to cease biologically harmful transmissions into your environment. You should mail your complaint to:

Federal Communications Commission

445 12th Street SW, Washington, DC 20554

People who typically have high radio frequency exposures are:

- Emergency service workers.
- Radio frequency technicians and engineers.
- Amateur radio operators.
- Utility metering workers.
- Roofers.
- People who live in communities that have Smart/AMR/AMI meters.
- People who work near to transmitter systems.
- People who are issued a radio transmitter in their jobs.
- People who work with RFID devices.
- People who work with wireless scanners.

Some reasonable health precautions are:

- Do not purchase wireless products.
- Shield the area of your home that has the utility meters near to it.
- Plant tall trees near to transmitting utility meters, as they will absorb the signal.

- Have the utilities remove their transmitting meters and replace them with non-transmitting versions.

- Do not live near to an antenna transmission system.

- Do not spend extended periods of time next to a transmitter.

- Avoid trips to scenic mountains that have transmitters on them. Generally these transmitters are the highest powered systems and the energy density will be very high in these locations.

- Avoid taking a job that is located near to a high powered transmitter.

- Avoid taking jobs that issue you with a radio transmitter for communications.

- Change you metal coil mattress to a foam one.

- Change your metal furniture to wooden furniture.

- Avoid being in areas with large numbers of people, as they may all have cellphones and WiFi devices. This increases the energy density.

- Avoid being inside metal structures with transmission devices. They will fill the area with reflected and interference energy.

If you combine the last two, you have an airplane! Frequent travelers are known to be amongst the sickest people in the general population.

You must remember that radiation transmitting antenna systems function by electrifying their environment. The peak energy density in the

environment is at the transmitter and it falls off with distance.

There are some systems that actually function as inadvertent transmission antenna systems:

- Electronic products.
- Home wiring.
- Electrical utility wiring.
- Earthing (grounding) systems.

The size of an antenna system is based on the frequency that it transmits at. For very low frequencies you have a very large antenna and for very high frequencies you have a very small antenna.

In the wireless radiation plague that we now find ourselves in, radio frequency (RF) meters have become popular products that people are obtaining to protect themselves. There are a few things that you should be aware of when operating these RF meters. When measuring radio frequency fields, the RF meter manuals typically instruct you to hold the meter at arms length. You should be aware that putting the RF meter near to metal can throw off the reading. That is why you should not put it near to electrical outlets.

Mass market RF meters are typically only accurate in the far field and the far field of residential transmitters can be very large at lower frequencies. Indeed I have a 400 MHz weather station transmitter at my home and you would have to keep the RF meter at least three feet away from that to get an accurate reading. My Tenmars TM-196 RF meter starts reading at 10 MHz which means that you would have to have the meter at least 30 meters away from a 10 MHz transmitting source to get an accurate reading!

Know the frequencies that you are dealing with and keep the minimum measuring distance at least one wavelength away from the transmitting device which is regarded as the near field. When measuring radio frequencies, the RF meters are typically only accurate in the far field which is outside of these distances:

- 1 MHz = 300 meters.
- 10 MHz = 30 meters.
- 50 MHZ = 6.0 meters.
- 100 MHz = 3.0 meters.
- 200 MHz = 1.5 meters.
- 300 MHz = 1.0 meter.
- 400 MHz = 0.75 meters.
- 500 MHz = 0.6 meters.
- 600 MHz = 0.5 meters.
- 700 MHz = 42.9 cm.
- 800 MHz = 37.5 cm.
- 900 MHz = 33.3 cm.
- 1.0 GHz = 30 cm.
- 2.0 GHz = 15 cm.
- 3.0 GHz = 10 cm.

- 4.0 GHz = 7.5 cm.
- 5.0 GHz = 6.0 cm.
- 10 GHz = 3.0 cm.

The health effects of the near field and far field exposures may be different. One is likely to be more toxic than the other. The near field contains far more energy than the far field. Regarding transmitter systems, generally it is the far field exposure that is quoted for the radiant power of the antenna system.

RADAR (RAdio Detection And Ranging) systems should be avoided. They have a very high powered pencil like beam of energy. The power can be in the range of 250,000 watts on the weather systems. RADAR workers have shown numerous health effects from near exposure to the beam. Cataracts are common in RADAR workers. If you live in a large city, you will be subjected to the RADAR from many RADAR systems. RADAR is in common use to open automatic doors on many shops and large buildings and they fill the area inside and outside of the shop with RADAR radiation. Some people may exhibit sickness when in a RADAR field. Dr. John Nash Ott filmed animals reacting to airport RADAR, they would react every time the sweep of the RADAR beam went through his home.

Male impotence is on the rise and so are the sales of impotence curing drugs. The impotence effect was noted to occur in RADAR workers during its development. Cell phones use RADAR frequencies, as does WiFi, and most domestic wireless products. It is likely that these wireless energies are contributing to the emasculation of the modern man.

Humans are acting as antenna systems and that is why you need to keep the RF meter away from you when performing measurements. Humans also act as reflectors and can increase the RF power density near to them.

Regarding electronic products, the operating frequencies have been getting very high due to the increasing computer processor speeds. If the product has not been designed well, then it may well be acting as a transmitter. An example of this is my digital television. It was transmitting energy that was stunting the growth of my outdoor plants over sixty feet away in the garden!

Electrical wiring is a horrendous transmitting device and you should pay attention to your home electrical system due to this. If you install certain products onto your electrical system, then you will turn it into a transmitting device! This effect has been especially noticed with people who use certain types of electronic energy star lighting products.

Electrical utility wiring is an interesting transmitter. The frequency of 60Hz is very low, but the utility transmission and distribution lines are very long, sometimes thousands of miles long! The utility companies may be inadvertently building transmitter systems. The city electrical distribution system may actually be a fractal antenna system! These are much smaller than conventional antenna systems. Harmonics on the utility power lines may make power lines that normally do not function as a transmitter turn into one.

Wikipedia states:

A fractal antenna is an antenna that uses a fractal, self-similar design to maximize the length, or increase the perimeter (on inside sections or the outer structure), of material that can receive or transmit electromagnetic radiation within a given total surface area or volume.

Because the electrical grounding system is connected to the utility neutral transformer connection, if the neutral conductor has dirty electricity on it, it may turn the entire area around your ground rods into a transmitter. The area for tens to hundreds of feet around your ground rods may turn into a transmission hot zone, even your plants may be acting as transmitters! Anyone in this area may get sick with extended exposure to this.

The AC electrical system operates in a range called the "Schumann Resonances" that are typically between 3 to 60 Hertz. Schumann resonances occur due to the cavity between the surface of the Earth and the conductive ionosphere, it acts as a "closed waveguide". Schumann resonances have distinct peaks at 7.86 Hz (fundamental), 14.3 Hz, 20.8 Hz, 27.3 Hz and 33.8 Hz. It does not surprise me to hear people saying that utility electrical frequencies affect them as it is likely that they are interfering with the natural Schumann resonances.

Due to these problems, I advise people to avoid transmitter systems, turn off the circuits in your home that you do not normally use, and to use minimal electronic products. Use mains filtering products with your electronic systems and also in the fuse board.

Metal should be avoided in the home and workplace because it acts as an absorber and reflector of radio frequencies and may distort the natural magnetic field. Avoid sleeping on metal coil mattresses as they have a wide range of unnatural energies flowing on them, you can easily obtain foam mattresses that do not have these problems. Unfortunately, some people may be developing electromagnetic hypersensitivity as they sleep! Use wooden chairs and wooden furniture as they are healthier.

Regarding wireless radiation exposures, the EMFields Acousticom 2 radio frequency meter manual states:

6 to 3 V/m: Too high for ambient levels.

1-0.3 V/m: Too high for many people.

0.1 to 0.05 V/m: Many people have symptoms.

0.02 to 0.01 V/m: Most people with EHS are okay.

I can recommend the free BioInitiative 2012 report for further reading on the subject of wireless radiation:

http://www.bioinitiative.org/

Books that document the known biologically harmful effects of wireless radiation are:

- "Disconnect" by Devra Davis.

- "Public Health SOS: The Shadow Side of the Wireless Revolution" by Magda Havas and Camilla Rees.

- "Cellular Telephone Russian Roulette" by Robert Kane.

The following pages show the side lobe effect and the many types of antenna systems that are commonly found today.

"The evidence for risks from prolonged cell phone and cordless phone use is quite strong when you look at people who have used these devices for 10 years or longer, and when they are used mainly on one side of the head. Recent studies that do not report increased risk of brain tumors and acoustic neuromas have not looked at heavy users, use over ten years or longer, and do not look at the part of the brain which would reasonably have exposure to produce a tumor."

Lennart Hardell, MD, PhD

Side lobe fields are around all directional transmitting antenna systems.

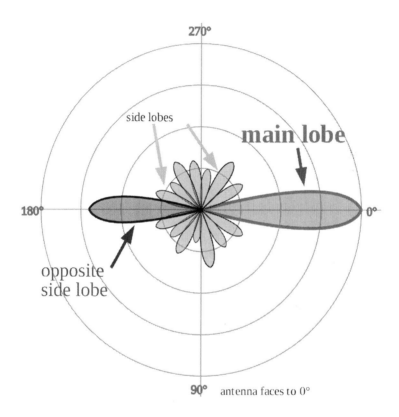

This extremely tall antenna system may be broadcasting very high power levels of electromagnetic radiation. The power poles and buildings give a sense to the height of this antenna system. Across the road is the local school.

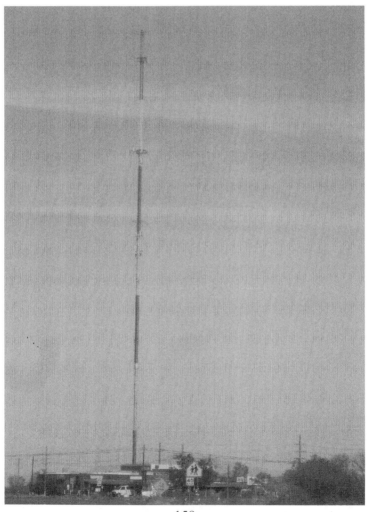

This is a typical dish antenna. Behind the wall is a residential neighborhood.

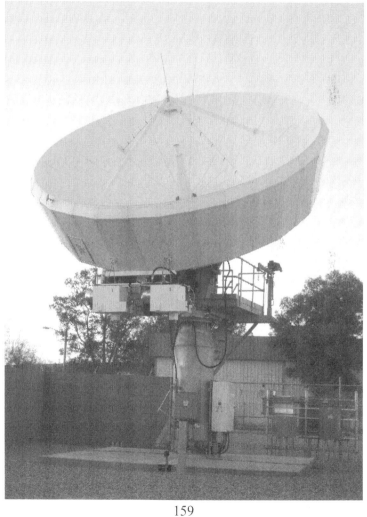

Here is a combined power distribution pole and antenna system. This was in front of the church in a residential neighborhood. At the back of the church was a playground.

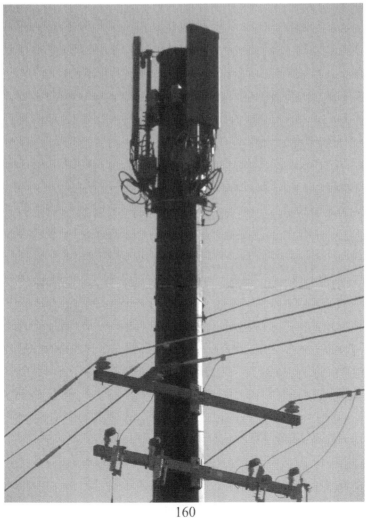

Here is a combined transmission line tower and antenna system. This was in the shopping mall.

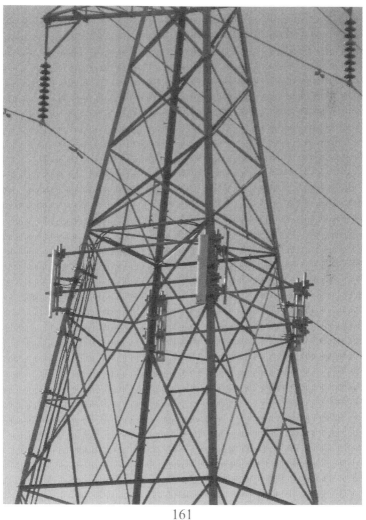

Here is a cell phone tower that is inappropriately sited. The wireless energy will be reflected from the electrical transmission lines. Both the transmission lines and the cell phone towers appear to be too close to the homes and the people may be sick in this location.

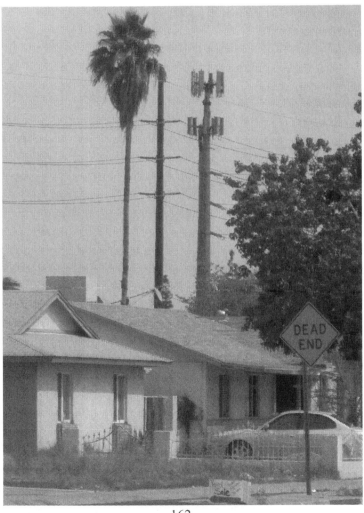

Here is a communications tower disguised as a palm tree. It was in the center of a residential area. These are called "stealth towers" in the industry.

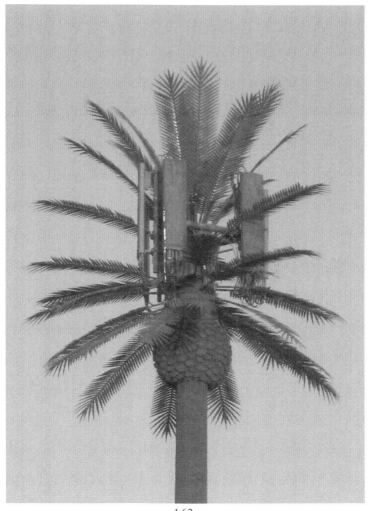

Antenna systems create solar radiation reflections and interference. They also create radio and microwave reflections and interference from other wireless transmission systems in the area. They short circuit the atmospheric layers that they pass through and may increase the rate of lightning strikes in the area if they are taller than the nearby surrounding structures.

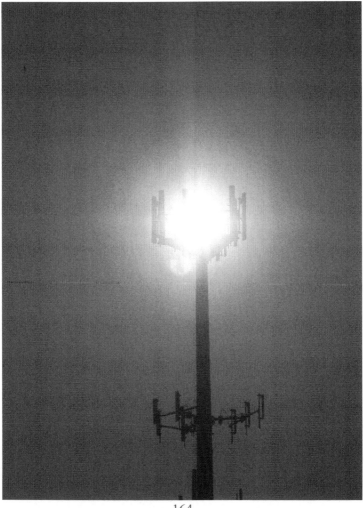

The police car may be a toxic environment today due to the extensive wireless communications in use, RADAR and LASER systems, the police computer system in the car, the flashing light emissions, and the car electromagnetic radiation emissions.

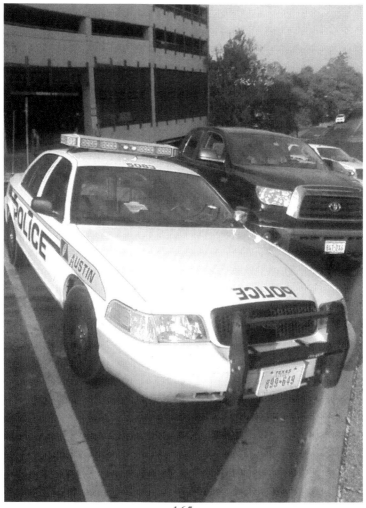

Satellites

Several decades ago the Earth only had one moon orbiting it. Today it has several thousand! The development of the Space industry has lead to massive amounts of satellites to be put in orbit. However, the Space industry did not do its homework prior to developing this field.

Mankind has known for thousands of years that when the moon eclipses the Sun, many strange behaviors are observed in animals and plants. All of the cycles go off and some plants will open their flowers and others will close them. The animal behaviors show a state of confusion. Some animals will wake up and others will go to sleep. Birds and bees stop flying. It does not matter what time of day the eclipse occurs, animal behavior is affected, so it is not just a change in lighting levels or heat that does this.

What an eclipse of the Sun does is to create a very strange radiation environment on Earth. The animals and plants are reacting to the changed electromagnetic radiation environment. Light and heat is just a small part of that changed environment.

The same effect appears to happen with satellites. The International Space Station is so large now, that it is the biggest thing in Space that can be photographed passing across the surface of the Sun, other than the moon. It is far larger than the sunspots! Every time a satellite passes in front of the Sun, the electromagnetic

environment is changed on the ground below. The effects of this are currently unknown.

However, in recent years a disorder in the Bees has shown up called "Bee Colony Collapse" disorder and it may well have a link to man-made satellite eclipses of the Sun that cause interference radiation to occur. Bee colony collapse was noted to significantly increase late in 2006, after the International Space Station had new solar arrays added onto it. The greatly increased its size and its effect when eclipsing the Sun.

The other problem with satellites is that they are continually bombarding the Earth with electromagnetic radiation! No one is quite sure what types of radiation that they are broadcasting as there are so many of them, many of which are secret military satellites. However, it is a fact that it is diverse.

This diverse man-made radiation is an addition of electromagnetic radiation on the surface of the Earth. Today, there is nowhere on the surface of the Earth that is free from it. The Earth has complete man-made satellite coverage.

These effects are shown in the next diagrams.

Satellite Interference

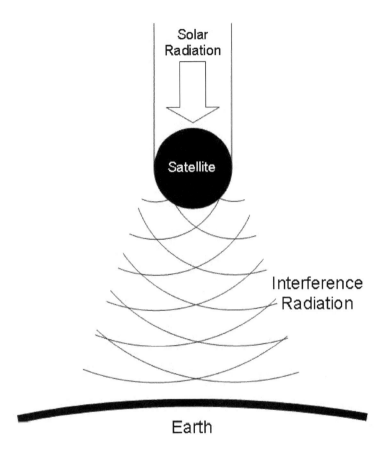

The Earth has complete artificial satellite coverage.

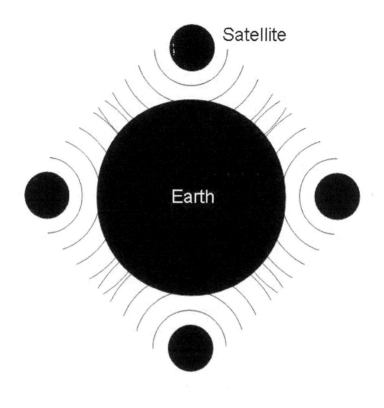

This is somewhat concerning, given the extensive denial about the health effects of electromagnetic interference. There is only one European country that appears to acknowledge it and that is Sweden. In Sweden, over 300,000 people are registered as having electromagnetic hypersensitivity. It clearly is a problem that is not unique to Sweden!

Unfortunately for the modern human, the development of the satellite industry took place without understanding these problems and today, it may actually be one of the biggest problems facing the future of humanity!

A scary thought about satellites is that once a nation has complete global coverage of the Earth, if they were to broadcast the correct types of electromagnetic radiation frequencies to the surface of the Earth, they could feasibly cause massive species extinction. This is called:

Satellite Extinction

Extinction energy frequencies are already being broadcast and they may be doing extensive harm to both plants and humans. The military has identified frequencies of energy that are harmful to human health and developed them for use in war zones. It is probably a feature that is present on secret military satellites.

I expect to see many countries in the future to be requesting the removal of satellites from their field of view of the sky. Satellites are the latest pollutant to be identified as a potential human health hazard.

"The U.S. spends over $2 trillion dollars on health care each year, of which about 78% is from people with chronic illnesses, without adequately exploring and understanding what factors—including EMF/RF— contribute to imbalances in peoples' bodies' in the first place. After reading The BioInitiative Report, it should come as no surprise to policymakers, given the continually increasing levels of EMF/RF exposures in our environment, that close to 50% of Americans now live with a chronic illness. I grieve for people who needlessly suffer these illnesses and hold out the hope that our government leaders will become more cognizant of the role electromagnetic factors are playing in disease, health care costs and the erosion of quality of life and productivity in America."

Camilla Rees, MBA

Power Lines

Power lines and poles running through the streets is a bad idea. They have a number of problems that may lead to illness:

- Electrostatic attraction.

- Electrostatic fields.

- Magnetic fields.

- Electric fields.

- Wide band radio wave emissions.

- Plasma emissions.

- Ion emissions.

- Ozone emissions.

- Nitrogen dioxide emissions.

- Reflection and interference of sunlight.

- Reflection and interference of radio and microwaves.

- AC electrification of the ground around them. (Stray voltage/current/frequency).

The utility power lines have setbacks that apply to them and for 13,800 volt AC lines, this setback is typically thirty feet either side of them. Building of homes and offices in these setbacks is generally not allowed due to the high electromagnetic fields that are present within the setback. The larger the voltage, the larger the

setbacks become. Power line set backs can be several hundred feet wide on the higher voltage transmission systems.

Power line wide band radio wave emissions may be erratic, occurring only at certain times of the day or during certain weather conditions. They are generally caused by the induction of electrical energy into the surrounding metalwork on the power pole that can cause sparks to jump between the metalwork. A failing or dirty insulator may have a similar effect. When a power line starts to emit radio waves, these may extend beyond the power line set back. The radio waves cannot be heard and a standard AM radio tuned to static (no radio station) can generally be used to detect them. Extended exposure to these wide band radio wave emissions may lead to electromagnetic hypersensitivity.

Power lines that carry harmonic energy may have a wide range of emissions from them. Harmonic energy levels will vary during the day and the seasons. It is important for human health to stay away from power lines that have harmonic energy on them.

While developing the power line section of this book, I spent three hours each night for two nights examining the power poles and power lines in the area of my home. I noticed the following conditions occurring over the following weeks:

- Headaches.
- Insomnia.

- Fatigue.

- Sore throat.

- Irregular heartbeats.

- Intestinal pains.

- General poor health.

- Heightened sexual desire occurred in the first few days after testing was finished, it appeared to be a side effect of electromagnetic interference withdrawal.

You should not spend time directly under power lines, as this will put you into the plasma field. Plasma is the fourth state of matter and under the power poles is an invisible flow of electrons from the power lines into the ground below.

There may be an electrostatic field present and this appears to be the reason why florescent tubes will light there. You can place 8 foot long florescent tubes vertically into the ground and watch them light up at night if the electrostatic field is present! A large piece of aluminum foil can also detect the electrostatic field with an AC voltage meter that has the ground probe electrically grounded. Do not touch the foil, as it may shock you! It may also damage your meter if the voltage on the foil is too large. It is a strange sensation to walk into a high powered electrostatic field as it is this field that makes your hair start to react. Nikola Tesla was trying to develop wireless lighting products using this field. We are fortunate that he never achieved his dream, as he may have made many people sick with his wireless lighting system. Nikola Tesla did end up being regarded as "nutty" and exposures to the electrostatic field may have been one of the things that was affecting him.

During my research into power lines producing AM radio frequencies, I noticed the reflection effect. The cell phone tower wireless energy seems to be interacting with the power lines and may be producing pockets of AM radio frequencies that can be picked up on a standard AM radio tuned to static (no radio station). If you were in one of these pockets for an extended time period, you may develop electromagnetic hypersensitivity.

You will find very high levels of body voltage around high voltage power lines and poles. It is shocking at how high they can get to. I will no longer work with high voltage systems due to the many problems that are around them and the strange behaviors that I have observed in people who work with it.

The following pages demonstrate the various effects of power lines.

Power lines and poles can have many types of large fields around them. "Dirty electricity" effects may cause extensive radio wave fields.

Power pole and power line emissions decay with distance

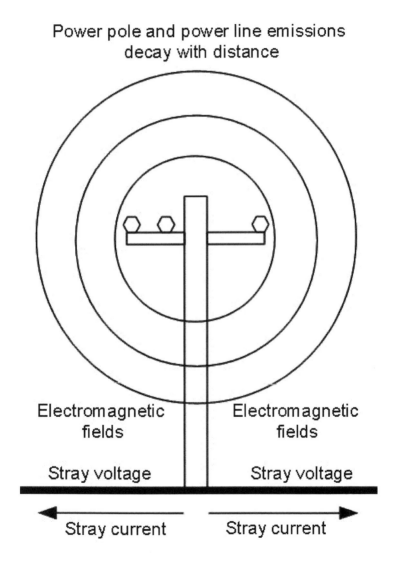

Electromagnetic fields

Electromagnetic fields

Stray voltage

Stray voltage

Stray current

Stray current

Induction effects in power pole metal work may cause sparks to jump between it which will cause radio wave emissions to occur. Defective insulators, oxidized clamps, defective fuses and damaged lightning arrestors may do the same.

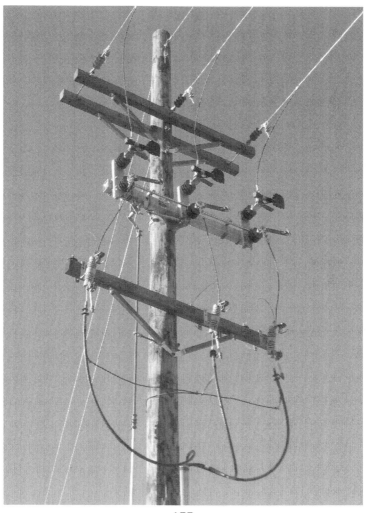

Power lines and poles can emit plasma and ions. The high voltage causes the electrostatic attraction effect. Power lines and poles have fields that extend out from the area that set backs should be applied to, to protect human health.

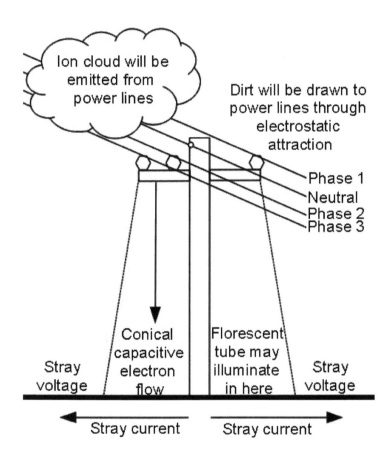

Power lines running down the pole may be the largest source of electromagnetic radiation in the human environment. You should stay away from poles that have conduits running down them.

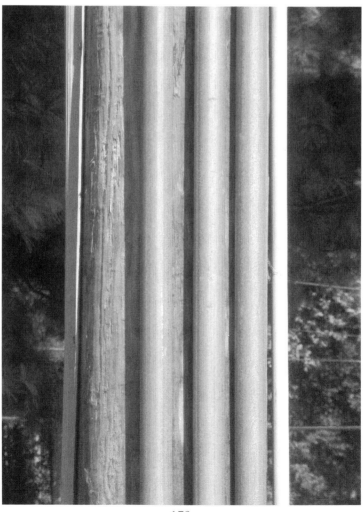

Power poles have a grounding (earthing) cable running down them. This connects the neutral cable at the top of the pole to the ground (earth) below. The ground in the vicinity of utility power poles is commonly electrified with stray voltage/frequencies and has ground currents in it.

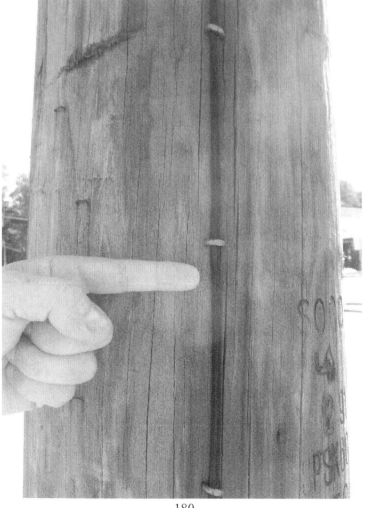

Power Line and Pole Solar Interference

The power poles and lines can interfere with the solar
radiation transmission when in front of the Sun.

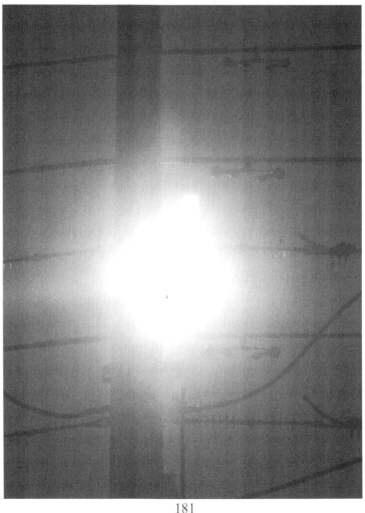

Power lines may cause solar, radio and microwave
reflections and interference effects to occur.

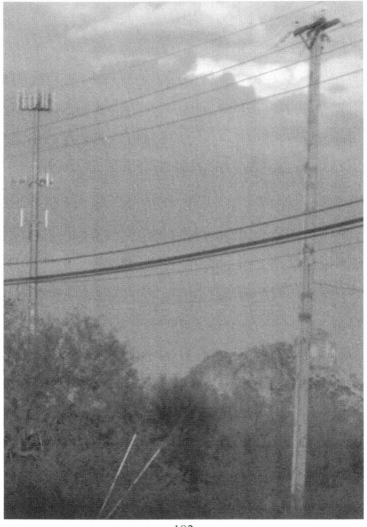

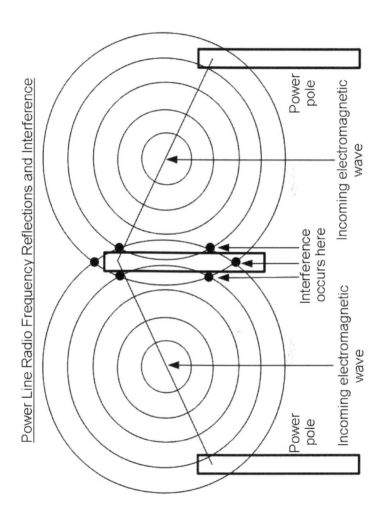

Power Line Radio Frequency Reflections and Interference

Power pole

Incoming electromagnetic wave

Interference occurs here

Incoming electromagnetic wave

Power pole

Incoming electromagnetic wave

Dr. Phillip Stoddard, Professor of Biological Sciences at Florida International University, has done extensive research on power lines. He has found very significant health risks from their presence:

- **The closer you live to a power line, the more likely you are to develop leukemia.**

- **Living in a magnetic field of 3.5 milli-gauss doubles the leukemia risk.**

- **Living within 0-50 meters of a power line doubles the risk of Alzhiemer's Disease and presents a 1.5 increased risk of developing senile dementia.**

- **Burying the power lines brings the magnetic fields closer.**

I do not recommend that you spend significant time underneath high voltage power lines, as you may be getting a free radiation treatment! They really should be fenced to keep people from venturing under them, especially young children. You should not buy a home that is underneath them if you value your health, as many people have become sick in such homes.

People have reported that they feel better in areas that the power lines are routed underground. However, this apparent improvement to health occurs only when the power lines are buried for at least half a mile in radius from the person. This is consistent with observations of lightning strikes preferring to hit tall grounded metallic objects. It is also consistent with the various electromagnetic emissions that power lines may create near to them.

A common problem on buried power lines is the corrosion of the concentric neutral. The concentric neutral is the wire that you see wrapped around the outside of the utility cable that comes down the power pole. If this corrodes, then the neutral starts to become high impedance and this will cause current to increase though the ground. Basically, corrosion of the concentric neutral will electrify the surrounding ground and is clearly a human health hazard. Faulty insulation on the live conductor that causes leakage currents will have a similar effect. Many children have been killed by stepping onto electrified ground during and after rains, when the problem is made much worse by conductive water.

The orientation of power lines with respect to the Earth's magnetic field may be an important factor in how they interact with human health. Power lines are known to interact with electromagnetic fields and this generally occurs during solar flare activity. Solar flares can knock out the electrical grid system if the flare is strong enough by inducing energy into the system. It appears that the electrical utilities may have built an inadvertent antenna system for solar flare energy!

It is not a good idea to live near to electrical equipment. The following locations should be avoided if you value your health:

• Streetlights.

- Power lines.

- Power poles.

- Transformers.

- Substations.

- Switch yards.

- Electrical power generation plants (coal, gas, oil, nuclear, steam, dams).

- Electronic power generation plants (wind, solar, tidal, wave, etc).

The areas in the vicinity of these may have large amounts of stray voltage/current/frequency.

Regarding human health, Wikipedia states:

*The UK Department of Health set up the Stakeholder Advisory Group on ELF EMFs (SAGE) to explore the implications and to make recommendations for a precautionary approach to power frequency electric and magnetic fields in light of any evidence of a link between EMF and childhood leukemia. The first interim assessment of this group was released in April 2007, and found that the link between proximity to power lines and childhood leukemia was sufficient to warrant a precautionary recommendation, including an option to **lay new power lines underground where possible and to prevent the building of new residential buildings within 60 m (197 ft) of existing power lines.** The latter of these options was not an official recommendation to government as the cost-benefit analysis based on the increased risk for childhood leukemia alone was considered insufficient to warrant it.*

The option was considered necessary for inclusion as, if found to be real, the weaker association with other health effects would make it worth implementing

Areas of known electromagnetic radiation hazards should be clearly signposted and preferably fenced to keep people out of harm. This is a particular problem for USA police officers and delivery drivers who spend their day driving around the city next to the power lines.

Areas around power plants may have strange environmental conditions associated with them. When reviewing the *Atmospheric Inversion Layers* article on bookrags.com, we find:

The mere presence of a city or factory often creates a microclimate of its own, creating a pocket of warm air within the cool ground layer. Smoke from a stack, instead of escaping upward or laterally, will descend to the ground, delivering a direct dose of pollution to residents of the area.

The following pictures demonstrate some of the problems.

Power plants emit large amounts of pollution, electromagnetic fields, and stray voltage/current/frequency effects. For this reason you should avoid living in areas that are near to power plants like this. The chimney emissions will cause solar radiation transmission problems.

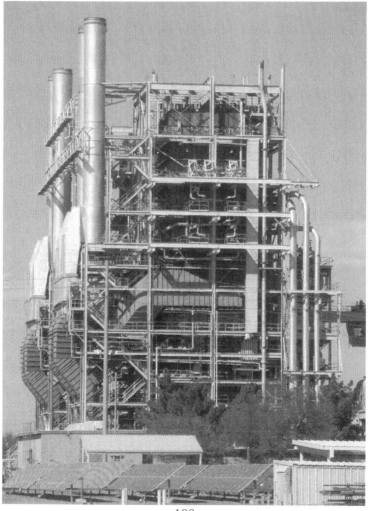

Utility switch yards should be avoided as there may be very large electromagnetic fields, electromagnetic reflections and interference, large ground currents, and stray voltage/frequencies in these areas.

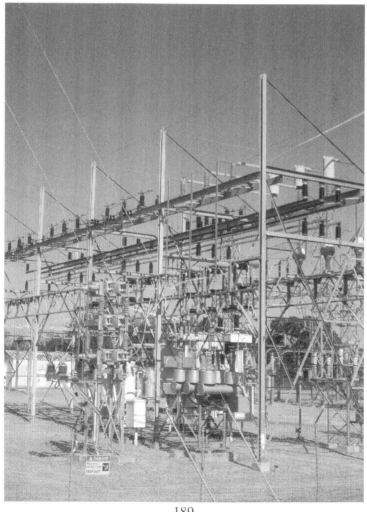

The lady in the picture has parked her car in the power line corridor and appears to be unaware of the detrimental health problems that may occur by spending extended time in this location.

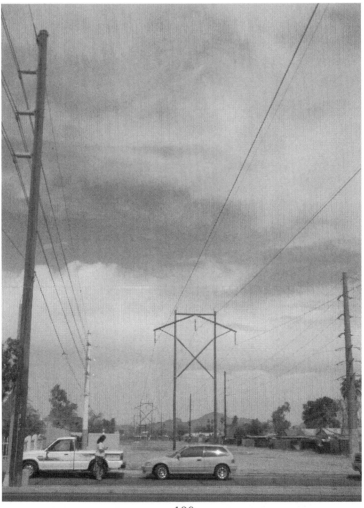

The USA commonly runs high voltage power lines along sidewalks and through residential areas. This lady appears unaware of the electromagnetic fields and stray voltage effects that may be present in her environment.

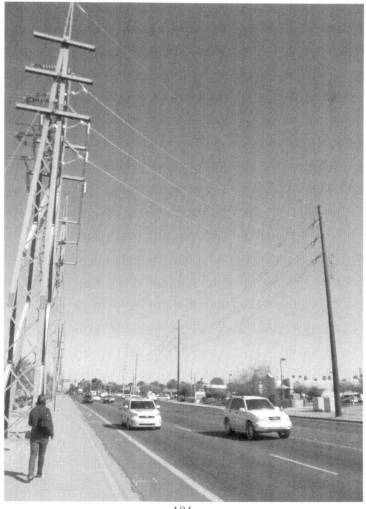

Around transformers you will find large electromagnetic fields and stray voltage/current/frequency at times. You should avoid spending time near transformers.

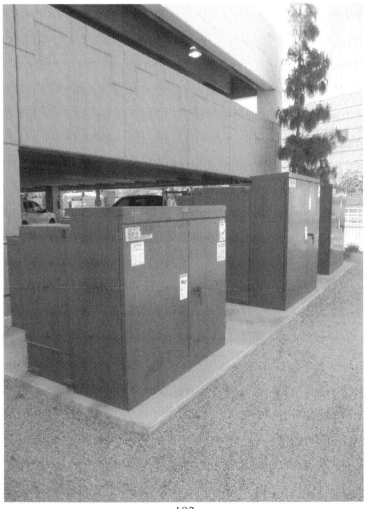

The sidewalk runs next to this equipment. The area should be fenced to keep people out of the electromagnetic fields. The other side of the wall should not be a human inhabited area to protect the health of the people in the building.

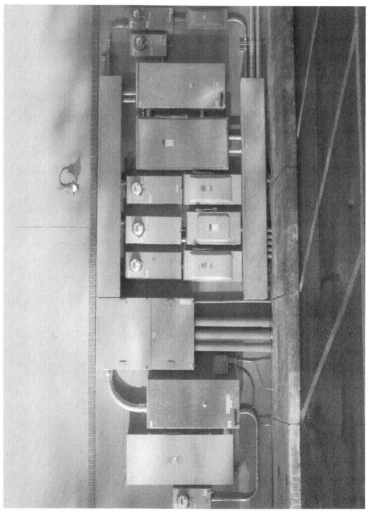

To put the public health system for electrical safety to the test to see what would happen, I reported a known defective utility electronic power plant that was generating high amounts of harmonic energy to these agencies:

- Occupational Safety & Health Administration (OSHA).
- State Public Commission (Utility company regulator).
- Federal Energy Regulatory Commission (FERC).
- North American Electric Reliability Corporation (NERC).
- Federal Communications Commission (FCC).

And this is what happened:

- OSHA said they investigated, found no problems, and shut down the complaint.
- State Public Commission never responded.
- FERC never responded.
- NERC said that it was the FCC's job.
- FCC responded and said that they would not investigate.

What I reported was a utility electronic power plant that was known to be producing extensive harmonics into the utility transmission system and that appeared to be affecting the health of the on site staff due to the excessive electromagnetic fields around the equipment. They were informed that I had developed classic symptoms of radio wave sickness while at the power plant and that I had observed similar symptoms in the on-site staff. They were also informed of extensive technical design mistakes and the dangerous problems that it was showing. This is what the FCC said about it:

Electric power transmission lines are considered "Incidental Radiators" under FCC Rules. See Title 47, Code of Federal Regulations, Section 15.3(n). [47 CFR §15.3(n)]. Incidental Radiators may be operated subject to the condition that no harmful interference is caused. See 47 CFR §15.5(b). ***FCC Rules prescribe no specific limits for the electric or magnetic fields radiated by Incidental Radiators.*** *The information that you supplied appears to suggest that you believe that interference may occur, but provides no evidence that interference is actually being caused.*

Because the FCC does not specifically limit emission levels from Incidental Radiators, no investigation can be initiated without a bona fide interference complaint. This office is aware of no complaints of harmful interference from the power plant.

The FCC does not regulate emissions or exposures at power line frequencies (typically 60 Hertz), which are classified as extremely low frequency (ELF). While harmonics of 60 Hz may be generated for various reasons, it is our believe that those harmonics exist at significant levels only up to a few kilohertz, and not into the radiofrequency (RF) regime. Some states and local jurisdictions have established their own requirements limiting ELF emissions or exposures in residential areas. I do not know whether any such limits exist in your area, but you may wish to contact the local planning department or state public utilities commission to find out. It is unlikely that such limits, if they exist, would apply to occupational settings however. I see that you have already contacted OSHA, which may have regulations that cover occupational exposure to ELF fields.

"Radio Wave Sickness" appears to be another term for a condition formerly known as Electromagnetic Hypersensitivity, having more recently been named Idiopathic Environmental Intolerance (IEI) attributed to electromagnetic fields. The World Health Organization notes that this "condition" has no agreed-upon diagnostic criteria and there is no consensus within the scientific community that its symptoms are linked to exposure to electromagnetic fields. Some information is available from the World Health

http://www.who.int/mediacentre/factsheets/fs296/en/index. html

The policy of the FCC with respect to environmental radiofrequency (RF) emissions has been developed to ensure that FCC-regulated sources do not expose the public or workers to levels of RF energy that are considered by expert organizations to be potentially harmful. The FCC has adopted guidelines for human exposure to RF electromagnetic fields based on recommendations from the U.S. Environmental Protection Agency (EPA), the Food and Drug Administration (FDA) and other federal health and safety agencies.

As you can see, there is an extensive web of deceit being woven within the governments agencies regarding harmful electrical electromagnetic radiation emissions into the human environment. They are clearly okay with workers health being damaged by dirty electricity and have been so for a very long time!

If you ever make a complaint about a known harmful electrical system, I wish you the best of luck...as you are going to need it!

"Electromagnetic fields are packets of energy that does not have any mass, and visible light is what we know best. X-rays are also electromagnetic fields, but they are more energetic than visible light. Our concern is for those electromagnetic fields that are less energetic than visible light, including those that are associated with electricity and those used for communications and in microwave ovens. The fields associated with electricity are commonly called "extremely low frequency" fields (ELF), while those used in communication and microwave ovens are called "radiofrequency" (RF) fields. Studies of people have shown that both ELF and RF exposures result in an increased risk of cancer, and that this occurs at intensities that are too low to cause tissue heating. Unfortunately, all of our exposure standards are based on the false assumption that there are no hazardous effects at intensities that do not cause tissue heating. Based on the existing science, many public health experts believe it is possible we will face an epidemic of cancers in the future resulting from uncontrolled use of cell phones and increased population exposure to WiFi and other wireless devices. Thus it is important that all of us, and especially children, restrict our use of cell phones, limit exposure to

background levels of Wi-Fi, and that government and industry discover ways in which to allow use of wireless devices without such elevated risk of serious disease. We need to educate decision-makers that 'business as usual' is unacceptable. The importance of this public health issue can not be underestimated."

David Carpenter, MD

<u>Home Electrical System</u>

The electrical power system in your home may also affect your health. Around electrical fuse boards there may be very high fields of microwave, radio, magnetic, electric, ion, and so on. The electromagnetic radiation emissions are a function of:

- The quality of the utility electricity.
- The quality of the utility electrical grounding system.
- The electrical equipment that is connected to the fuse board.
- Smart/AMR/AMI transmitting utility meters.
- The type of structure that it is mounted to.
- The quality of the home electrical grounding system.
- The construction of the electrical fuse board.
- The routing of the cables that connect to the equipment.
- The presence of an alternate energy system (such as solar photovoltaic or wind).
- The distance to the utility transformer.

It may be possible that Leukemia in children is linked to the location of the fuse board and the electrical meter on the home. The health of children is a particular concern with the advent of Smart/AMR/AMI utility

meters, as they broadcast radio frequencies into their surrounding environment. Babies and children are the ones who are most affected by these effects.

Some fuse boards may need filters installing and line terminators on their radial circuits. These are important in areas that have electrical power quality issues (Dirty electricity).

A simple filtering circuit is shown in the next few pages that can help with reducing dirty electricity. It is simply a selection of different size capacitors that are connected in parallel at the fuse board. The capacitor plates are all different sizes in order to filter different frequencies that may be present on the AC system.

The simple filter should assist with reducing radio frequencies present at the fuse board. It should be mounted in a metal enclosure, as it will be radiating radio frequencies if it is filtering them from the utility network. The filter uses negligible power. If it starts to buzz, then you will likely have a frequency problem that your electrician will need to diagnose.

The location considerations for electrical fuse boards and associated equipment are also shown in the following pictures.

"Sensitivity to electromagnetic radiation is the emerging health problem of the 21st century. It is imperative health practitioners, governments, schools and parents

*learn more about it. **The human health stakes are significant.***"

William Rea, MD

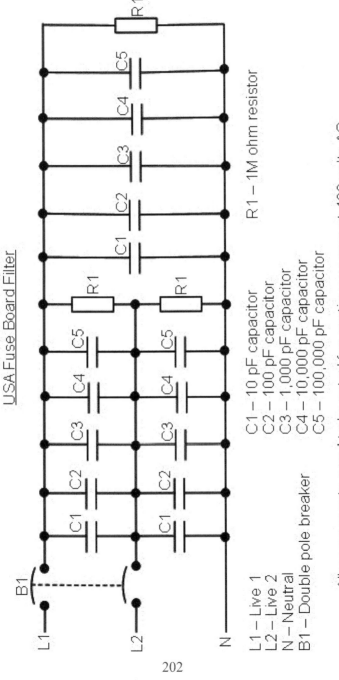

USA Fuse Board Filter

R1 – 1M ohm resistor

C1 – 10 pF capacitor
C2 – 100 pF capacitor
C3 – 1,000 pF capacitor
C4 – 10,000 pF capacitor
C5 – 100,000 pF capacitor

L1 – Live 1
L2 – Live 2
N – Neutral
B1 – Double pole breaker

All components need to be rated for continuous use at 400 volts AC

202

USA Fuse Board Filter

This is what the USA fuse board filter looks like when it is built.

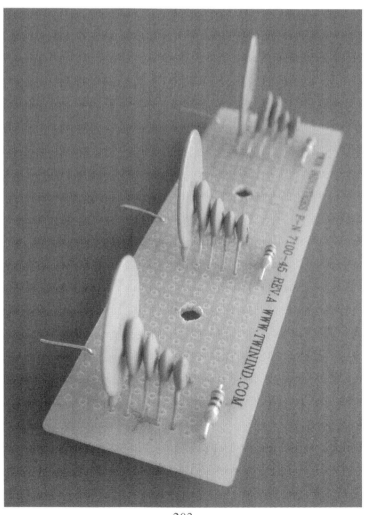

European Fuse Board Filter

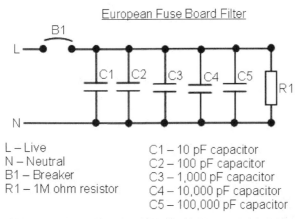

L – Live
N – Neutral
B1 – Breaker
R1 – 1M ohm resistor

C1 – 10 pF capacitor
C2 – 100 pF capacitor
C3 – 1,000 pF capacitor
C4 – 10,000 pF capacitor
C5 – 100,000 pF capacitor

All components need to be rated for continuous use at 400 volts AC

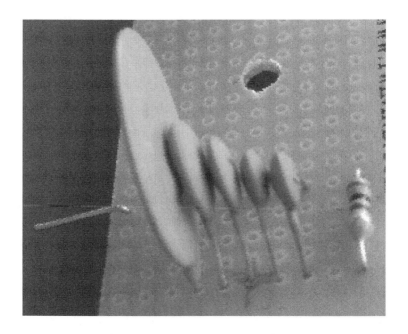

A simple capacitive filter can be made using a resistor in parallel with a capacitor connected to the live and neutral electrical plug connections.

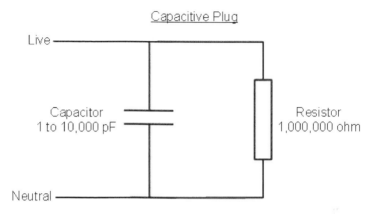

Capacitive Plug

All components are to be rated for continuous use at the electrical system AC voltage. You may need to insert a fuse on the live connection, depending on your electrical system. Reduce the size of the capacitor if it causes interference with other equipment on the circuit. It buzzes when it is filtering high frequencies from the electrical system.

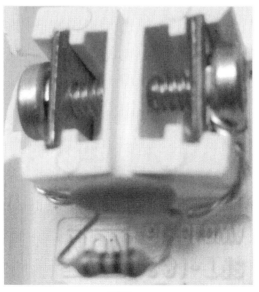

Electrical fuse boards should not be mounted in human habitation areas due to the fields that extend out from them and the possible radio frequency transmissions. An ideal location is on the side of the garage.

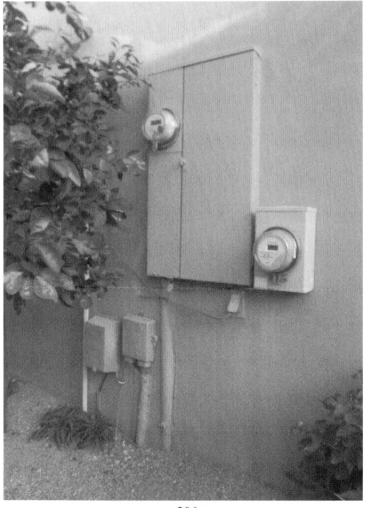

Unfortunately, the fuse board in the previous picture was located directly behind the master bed! Electrical fuse boards should not be mounted on human habitations.

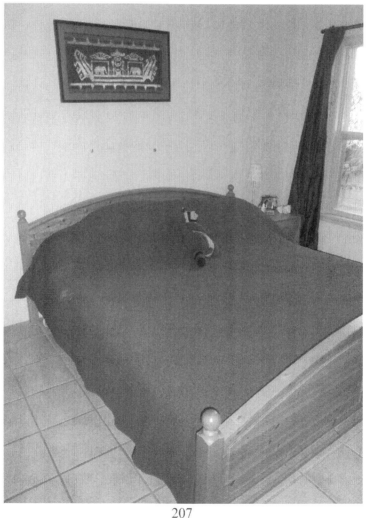

When living in apartments, it is preferable not to live in the apartment that has the electrical meters on the wall. There will be high electromagnetic fields in this area and possibly radio frequency emissions.

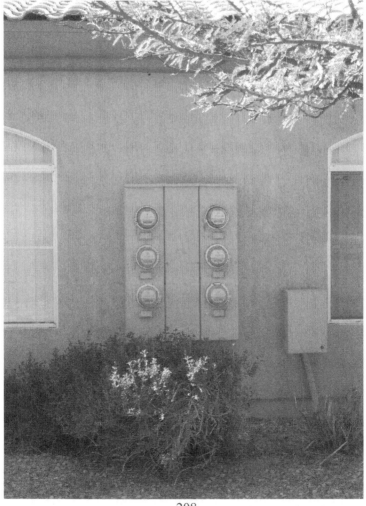

The electromagnetic fields around solar photovoltaic systems can vary with the sunlight. You may find the fields entering the human environment below.

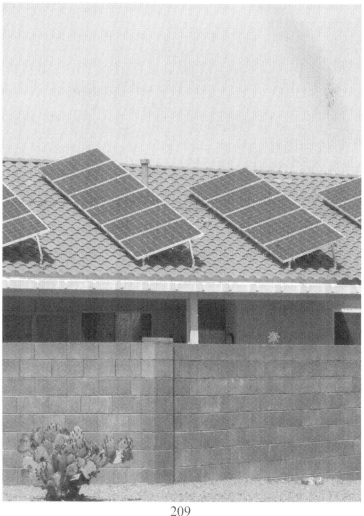

Earthing

The utility supplies a combined earth (ground) and neutral connection to your home that splits into the earth (ground) and neutral connection at your fuse board. The ground rods that you see near fuse boards are to effectively connect this combined earth and neutral cable to the ground potential of the property.

The earth and neutral connections will float up and down in proportion to the load on the distribution system in your area if it is not grounded properly by both the utility and the homeowner. The human body cannot sense low AC voltages, currents nor frequencies on the earthing (grounding) system and you may slowly get sick with prolonged exposure to it.

You should remember that the electrical earth (ground) connection in your home or office connects directly to the neutral transformer winding connection that is supplying the electricity. It may be carrying an AC voltage!

This is shown in the next diagram.

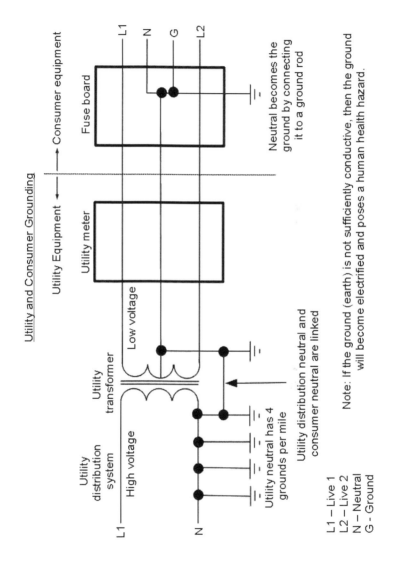

Utility and Consumer Grounding

Consumer equipment

Utility Equipment

L1
N
G
L2

Fuse board

Neutral becomes the ground by connecting it to a ground rod

Utility meter

Low voltage

Utility transformer

Utility distribution system

High voltage

Utility neutral has 4 grounds per mile

Utility distribution neutral and consumer neutral are linked

L1

N

L1 – Live 1
L2 – Live 2
N – Neutral
G - Ground

Note: If the ground (earth) is not sufficiently conductive, then the ground will become electrified and poses a human health hazard.

During researching electrical grounding systems, it became apparent that many grounding systems are actually acting as antenna systems for wireless energy. The wireless energy is very low at the ground rods, but as you move further away from the ground rods, you start finding increasing wireless energies on the home ground wiring. Indeed, Nikola Tesla documented that antenna systems are more efficient when connected to a ground rod! As such, you should be aware that any cable connected to a ground rod becomes a receiver for wireless energy. The longer that cable is, the more wireless energy that you will find on it.

The concept of grounding is quite interesting. The electrical system was originally designed to be a one wire supply system with an earth return through grounding rods. It was only when people started to get shocked by the electrified earth that a return wire was also installed, which we now call the neutral. However, the ground rods remained and if the neutral is higher in voltage potential than the ground, then it will feed AC voltage and current into the ground. In other words, the ground rods electrify the ground with AC electricity! This is a particular problem anywhere where the ground is a poor conductor of electricity, such as the desert southwest USA.

This is shown in the next diagram.

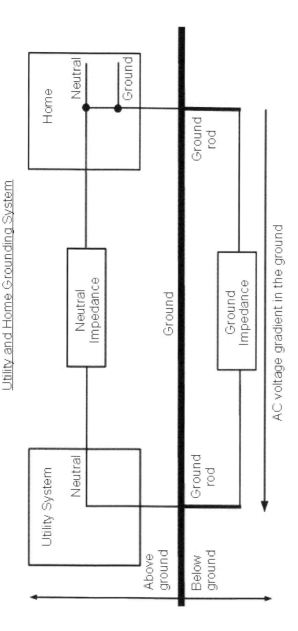

Utility and Home Grounding System

The ratio of the neutral to ground impedance determines the current flowing in the neutral cable and through the ground (earth). If the ground impedance is high, then all current will flow on the neutral cable and raise the voltage on the ground rods. This may create excessive stray voltage that can affect peoples health.

When reviewing the BBC News article *Louis Theroux on dementia: The capital of the forgetful,* we find:

For years Phoenix has been a mecca for America's elderly, who are attracted by the year-round sun and dry desert heat. Now increasingly it is a kind of capital of the forgetful and the confused.

One has to wonder if stray voltage/current/frequency is causing some of their problems? The dry desert of the southwest USA is one of the poorest conductors of electricity that you will find. Effective grounding systems need water in the ground to increase the conductivity of it. Due to this, grounding systems vary in their effectiveness due to the seasonal water content of the ground.

You should be aware that anywhere that a ground rod is installed, that there may be AC voltage/current/frequency in the vicinity of it. The electrification of the earth may extend several hundred feet from the ground rods. You should keep your shoes on and keep children and pets away from these areas. AC electrification of the earth commonly occurs around streetlights, pad mounted transformers, power poles and lines, and electrical substations too! People who walk their dogs are at particular risk from these energized earth effects.

This is shown in the next diagram.

Electrical Grounding System

Top View

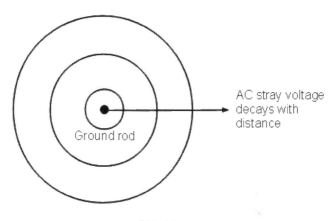

Side View

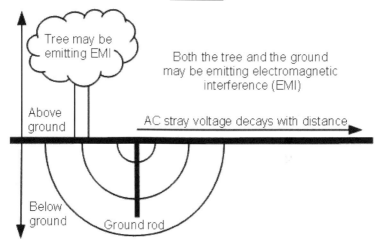

The Ufer ground uses a concrete encased electrode and is a particular problem, as it generally uses the foundation of the building to get the ground connection. This means that the stray voltage peaks near to where it is installed. At my home, this area is the garage floor that is next to my kitchen tiled flooring. As such, there is a significant AC voltage on these floors at certain times of the day!

You should avoid wearing leather soled shoes, as these will connect you into stray voltage sources. Your shoes should have insulated soles in areas that have electricity. Do not walk around barefoot in environments that have electricity installed into them!

A utility electrical substation is shown in the next diagram. The substation relies on an earth (ground) return path for the electricity and as such, the area around electrical substations may have large amounts of electrical ground currents and stray voltage/frequency present.

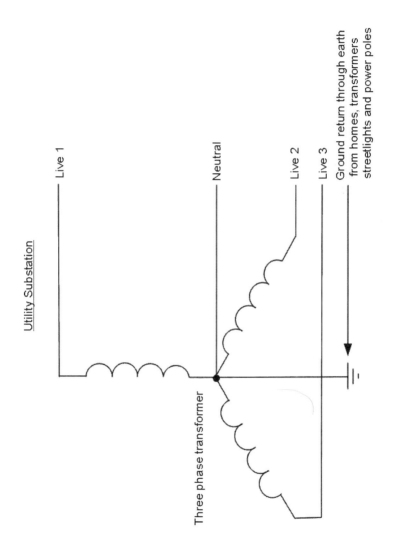

Grounding electrical and plumbing systems at the home can create voltages in the home that are commonly referred to as "stray voltage". Stray voltage is a well known effect in the diary industry and it can wreak havoc on the health of farmers, their families, and their livestock. As one farmer reports:

"It's a slow, painful tortuous death, is what it is for them," said Siewert, who with his father, Harlan, owns Siewert Holsteins in Zumbro Falls. "It's like watching someone die of AIDS."

One of the things that has caused stray voltage/current/frequency to become prevalent in the human environment is the widespread adoption of plastic services to houses. In the past, the plumbing was cast iron drains, galvanized steel supply pipes, and copper tubing. All of these were relatively good conductors of electricity and supplied good grounding to the home. This has changed and plumbing is now commonly plastic, which is an insulator to electricity.

You can get a sense to how biologically toxic an electrical grounding system is by grounding the pot of a Dieffenbachia (Dumb Cane) plant to the electrical system ground connection. I have done this and I obtained a "Frankenstien" plant that is very tall and deformed compared to my controls. It takes several months of growth to obtain such a deformed plant. This is shown in the next picture.

My "Frankenstein" electrical utility grounded soil, stray voltage/current/frequency exposed Dieffenbachia plant grew very tall with an unusual double canopy of miniature leaves that are distinctly different from each other. This growth pattern is unique to this plant and it is the tallest Dieffenbachia in my home at 18 inches from the soil surface to the top leaf tip.

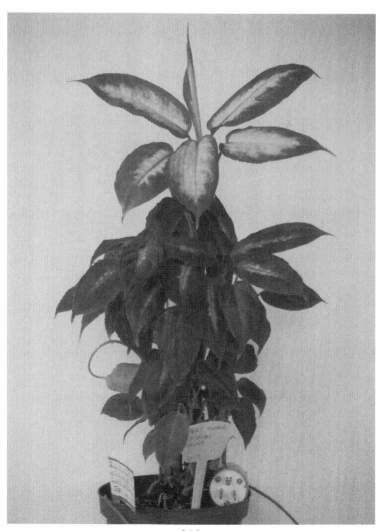

The stray voltage effects are shown on the following pages, as measured in the evening at my home during September 2011 in Arizona, USA. The Amprobe 5XP-A meter is logging the minimum and maximum vales of the voltage on the electrical grounding system. The measurements in the garden were also performed with the Amprobe 5XP-A meter. As you can see, there is an AC voltage gradient from the electrical ground rods at the front of the home to the back of the home where the reference ground rod is installed. The reference ground rod is installed well away from the home and electrical systems. There are no electrical connections to it.

The Amprobe 5XP-A multimeter is logging voltage values of the electrical outlet ground pin (Right probe) to the garden ground at the back of the home (Left probe).

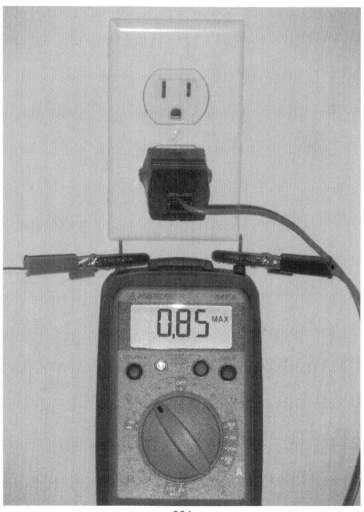

Garden Stray Voltage

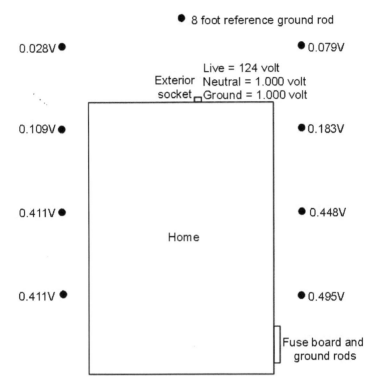

Stray voltage measurements in the garden using an
Amprobe 5XP-A multimeter. As can be seen, there is a
voltage gradient through the property.

During logging the utility ground to the garden ground for current and voltage in August and September 2011, these are the range of values that I recorded at my home:

- 0.07 to 1.66 volts.

- 2.7 to 55 milli-amps.

- 60 Hertz.

- Low values occurred near sunrise, high values occurred between 16:00 to 20:00 mid-week.

- The electrical distribution system had high loads due to air conditioning loads running in the summer heat.

It is interesting to note that for electrocution to occur in water, the following conditions must exist:

- **Assuming a wet human body impedance of 300 ohms.**

- **Muscle control in the human is lost at between 6 to 30 milli-amps.**

- **1.8 to 9 volts of 60 Hertz AC is needed.**

As we can see, the conditions at my home are very close to those required for a water electrocution. If a surge from an electrical fault or lightning strike on the utility system occurred, then the conditions for a water electrocution may occur. I would be very concerned if I owned a swimming pool!

Plastic plumbing may be hazardous to human health, as it
does not ground the water contained within the pipes. As
such, any plastic plumbing that is routed with electrical
cables may start to couple into the fields of the cables. The
result is the water may become electrified. You may well
end up with stray voltage/current/frequency at your faucets,
basins, showers and bathtubs! Clearly an undesirable
effect.

**Copper plumbing may have stray
voltage/current/frequency on it if your grounding
system is bad. You may want to install a dielectric
isolator after the electrical ground in order to prevent
the pipes from being electrified within the home with
AC stray voltage/current/frequency. Many people have
reported that their health significantly improved after
doing this. You will need to consult with a qualified
electrician about this.**

If your walls are conductive, then you may find that your
walls are electrified with stray voltage/current/frequency as
well as your flooring. This may occur in a brick home or
metal framed home. It may also occur when the walls are
wet after rain. You may find an AC voltage gradient in
them that is similar to what you find around the ground
rods. The use of metal back boxes for the electrical sockets
and switches may increase this effect.

This is shown in the next diagram.

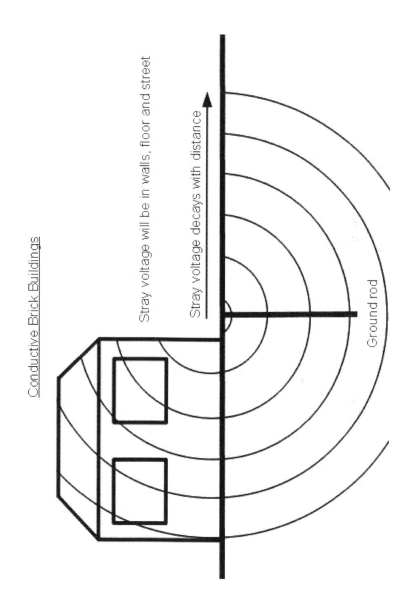

Conductive Brick Buildings

Stray voltage will be in walls, floor and street

Stray voltage decays with distance

Ground rod

Stray voltage/current/frequency in the past was commonly associated with swimming pools and hot tubs, but is now rapidly becoming prevalent in many other areas throughout modern society. Have you ever wondered why competent swimmers drown in their own swimming pools? It may well be stray current that killed them, particularly if an electrical fault or lightning strike occurred in the area. Electricity easily couples into water systems and electrifies the water.

Antistatic devices (ASD) are commonly used in many industries and may present a health hazard to those who work with these. If they are connected into a poor quality grounding system, then they may well cause an AC voltage and many frequencies to appear on the human body. My research into this area is indicating that a direct long term exposure to a low level AC voltage that contains many frequencies may cause the human body to slowly fall into illness and perhaps onto disease. It matches the findings of the diary industry that just 0.5 volt of AC electricity exposure can lead to illness in the human body. The effects that I noticed during two weeks of wearing an antistatic strap that was connected to the electrical utility ground were:

- Headaches.
- Insomnia.
- Fatigue.
- Irregular heartbeats.

It was easily cured by removing the antistatic strap. The symptoms cleared up within a few weeks. When I investigated the grounding system I found 1.5 volts of AC electricity on it when compared to the garden and a wide range of frequencies extending into the megahertz range!

Antistatic equipment is common in the hospital operating room. Dr. William Rae determined that his allergic and neurological symptoms were caused by the electromagnetic fields in the operating room. He subsequently discovered that he was not alone in his electromagnetic hypersensitivity, and that there was a growing population of patients with the same condition. These people are typically told by their physicians that their symptoms are "all in their minds" and that they should seek psychiatric care.

Surgeons have been noticed to be a group of the population that suffer from addictions, depression, and burning out. It appears to be much worse in the female surgeons and this matches the findings that the female body is more sensitive to the effects of AC electricity.

You should avoid using antistatic devices in areas that are known to be electrified. You may find a significant AC voltage waveform appearing on it from time to time!

Whether you use an antistatic device or not, you may find yourself connected into the AC supply through your environment. Walking around in your bare feet or socks on conductive flooring, such as tile or outdoors, may expose you to an AC voltage. Believe it or not, walking the dog may expose you to AC voltage through the dog lead if it is conductive!

Using any device that has a metal case and is electrically grounded through the cable may expose you to an AC voltage. Metal sewing machines, metal mobile homes, metal appliances, and metal electric power tools can be examples of this. Anything that is conductive and electrically grounded that humans come into contact with is a potential health risk. Keeping your shoes on can reduce the risk, as can wearing electrically insulated gloves.

Stray voltage/current/frequency can be on your sewer system and it can come up through the toilet, shower, bath, and sink drains. It is difficult to avoid from these locations and it is recommended that you do not urinate into electrified toilets. Connecting into an electrical source through your urine stream should be expected to lead to long term internal health problems.

Plants can be affected by stray voltage and they may show stunted growth, deformed growth, or go dormant. In extreme cases they may die.

The extensive testing that I have performed showed that a direct contact exposure to the AC electrical system is far more biologically toxic than an indirect exposure through the air. The body appears to have an increased ability to tolerate the air induced exposure that is not present with direct contact with stray voltage/current/frequency from the electrical ground.

Stray voltage/current/frequency varies with the time of the day and can significantly change. Early in the morning it can be very low and during the peak electrical load periods, it can be very high. A multimeter with a minimum and maximum logging feature is ideal to find the range of values of stray voltage and current. I have found the Amprobe 5XP-A multimeter to be ideal for this purpose, as it has a 16 day battery life when using a 9 volt alkaline battery. To get the highest accuracy reading of stray voltage and current, you should be using an oscilloscope, as the voltage and current waveform may be highly distorted. Using a time lapse camera will allow you to record the waveform over long periods of time.

The voltage waveform on the grounding system in my home is shown in the next picture. This was measured at the grounding pin in the home at the electrical outlet. The measurement was taken at 19:30 on a Saturday night after it had just gone dark on April 28th, 2012. It was a warm night and most people were not running their air conditioning units.

You should remember that anything that has a metal case that is grounded will have this voltage on it, such as stainless steel appliances. An antistatic device (ASD) that was plugged into the wall outlet would also have this voltage on it. A similar voltage would also be on electrically conductive tiled and concrete flooring near to the ground rods.

The frequency content of the voltage waveform is shown in the following pictures. You can see that there are a wide range of frequencies on the grounding system.

The distorted voltage waveform on the grounding system of my home. It is almost two volts peak to peak. It is much higher in summertime!

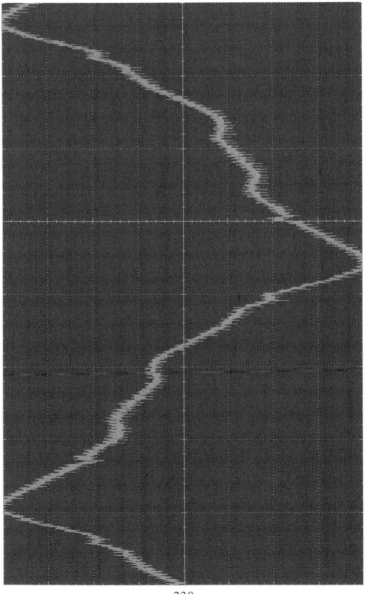

The low frequency content on the grounding system. The repeating 60 Hz harmonics can clearly be seen.

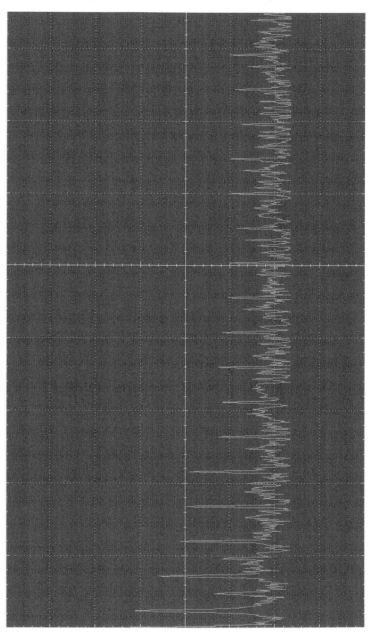

The high frequency content on the grounding system. A peak can clearly be seen centered around 1,250,000 Hz.

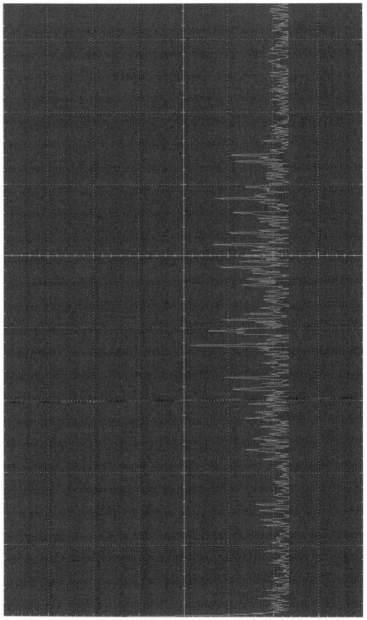

You can sometimes pick up the frequencies coming off grounding systems using a standard AM radio tuned into static (no radio station). If you put the radio near to the grounding system, you may hear it start buzzing. A telephone voice coil used to record telephone calls connected into an amplified speaker can be used to detect the lower frequencies on grounding systems. Radio Shack sells the voice coils, they are called "Recorder Telephone Pickup" Model: 44-533, Catalog #: 44-533.

Communities that have alternate energy systems in them may have large amounts of frequency content on the grounding systems that come from electronic power generation systems that are called "inverters". The next images show the voltage and frequency content of a neighborhood with a large amount of solar photovoltaic generation systems installed into it. The ground voltage measurement is highly distorted and will be producing harmonics. It has approximately 1.2 volts peak to peak and a 60Hz waveform. The ground frequency scale goes from 0Hz at the bottom of the page to 500,000Hz at the top of the page. There are significant frequency spikes present in this range. This will typically change during the day, as it will vary with the sunlight.

Solar PV Powered Neighborhood Ground Voltage

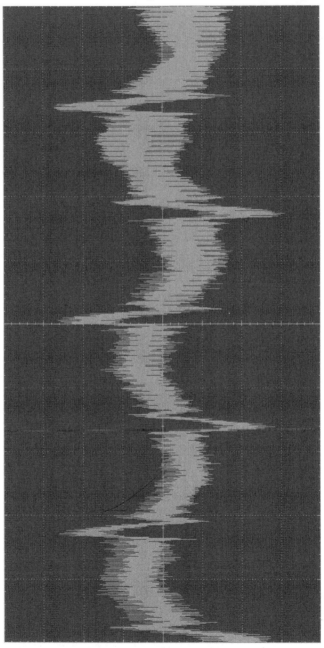

Solar PV Powered Neighborhood Ground Frequency

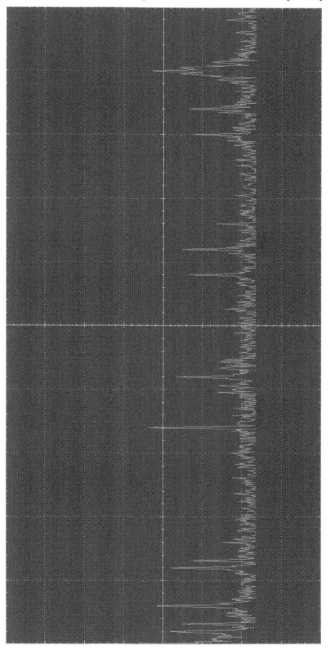

Whether you like it or not, stray voltage/current/frequency is present within your own body. The body will couple into electromagnetic fields and this can be detected with a digital multimeter or an oscilloscope. The alternating current voltage of the human body can get quite high, often exceeding fifteen volts when next to an AC cable. Just 0.5 volt of stray AC voltage is known to affect animals and just 2 volts of AC voltage is known to kill them with long term exposure! The farming industry has set an upper limit on stray voltage of 0.5 volt AC due to the effects that have been observed in the animals.

The electrical grounding system on my home in August and September 2011 regularly exceeded this value by three times the allowable animal contact value! I have noticed sore knees and aching bones occurring every year in summertime at my current home which I now have linked to this stray voltage/current/frequency effect. I no longer walk around the home in bare feet, I wear insulated slippers now.

Ground loops can be a particular problem. They occur where there are multiple ground (earth) paths for the electricity to take. It is commonly seen to occur on metal pipework. You may find very high magnetic fields around such pipework from the current flow through it. It can be prevented by having a licensed contractor install dielectric isolators into the pipework.

Ground loops can also occur from appliances that have metal feet. The metal feet provide a current path through the conductive floor to the ground (earth). It can be prevented by having insulated plastic feet on the appliances. If you encounter this, simply put insulated plastic spacers under the metal appliance feet to break the ground loop. Many people have found that their health problems subside by taking this simple action.

High magnetic fields may occur on electrical wiring when the neutrals from multiple electrical circuits have been inadvertently connected together in the home. They can also occur if the neutral has short circuited to the ground. Instead of the neutral current flowing down the same cable as the live current, it takes an alternate path that creates a current imbalance in the electrical cables that creates high magnetic field emissions.

The characteristics that are observed in animals that have been exposed to stray voltage/current/frequency are:

- Reduced feed and water intakes.
- Increased defecation in the milking parlor.
- Increased incidences of mastitis.
- Elevated somatic cell counts (white blood cells in the milk).
- Increased still births.
- Calves born crippled.
- Calves born blind.
- Sickly newborn calves.
- Calves dying within several days of birth.
- Crippled cows.
- Joint problems.
- Behavioral changes.

- Anxiety.
- Nervousness.
- Fatigue.
- Depression.
- Poor hair coats.
- Poor reproductive performance.
- Increased aborted pregnancies.
- Reduction in milk output.
- Depressed immune systems.
- Increased death rates.

In the human, the effects appear to be similar:

- Changed personality.
- Degrading mental health.
- Forgetfulness.
- Anger.
- Irritability.
- Anxiety.
- Fatigue.
- Eye problems.
- Nerve tingling.
- Itchy skin.
- Joint problems, especially the hips, knees and ankles.

- Arthritis symptoms.

- Aching bones.

- Sexual problems.

- Suicide.

- The problems may appear to be seasonal or related to the time of day.

- Cancer, Fibromyalgia, and Chronic Fatigue Syndrome are suspected to be linked to it.

So how do you prevent stray voltage/current/frequency from occurring? Here are some suggestions:

- Install your ground rods well away from your home and use insulated cable ran inside plastic conduit to connect them to your fuse board.

- Landscape the area that your ground rods are located in to prevent people from walking and sitting on the ground in that area.

- Get the utility to install a stray voltage isolator onto the transformer that feeds your property.

- Have the utility install larger neutral cables to your property.

- Have the utility provide you with a separate ground cable from the transformer.

- Have a licensed contractor install dielectric unions in areas that have ground loops occurring.

Ultimately, the electrical utility system should never have connected energized conductors into the ground. It was just a really bad decision that was made before the stray voltage/current/frequency problem was discovered in the 1970's. Instead of doing the right thing when the utility industry became aware of it, it has been in constant denial by them ever since. They know that this effect is ruining peoples lives and they are okay with that. Willfully polluting the ground with AC electricity is just another aspect of how the electrical utility companies will be remembered by the next generation.

This quote by Russ Allen, author of "Electrocution of America", sums up how stray voltage has been allowed to become the problem that it is today:

"Utilities are rarely fined for their wrongdoings. What's more, they have nobody inspecting their distribution systems—they regulate themselves. Utility companies have polluted our water, our air and the soil we walk on. The effect on farms and livestock alone is enough to warrant mass concern, but factor in what it does to people, and you have a huge crisis on your hands."

Russ Allen

Stray Voltage, Stray Current and Stray Frequency

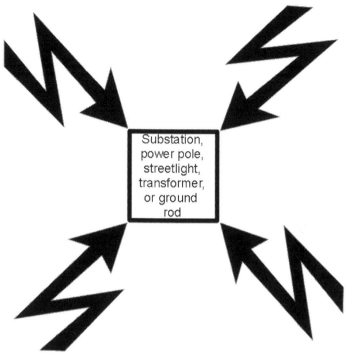

The earth around electrical equipment is commonly electrified by ground rods. You should avoid coming into contact with electrified earth, as it is a human health hazard. You should keep children away from these areas.

DC and AC

The direct current (DC) system is either positive or negative polarity and does not use the sine waves and frequency of the alternating current (AC) system. It simply supplies a fixed voltage all of the time. Batteries are a form of DC electricity and most people associate them with the DC system.

It is clear why the alternating current (AC) system was chosen over the direct current (DC) system. One word sums it up:

Fire

The DC system suffers from arcing and fires. We know this due to the recent adoption of DC solar power systems for power generation. As they are aging, people are finding that they are failing through arcing, and in some cases, going on fire. Once DC has started to arc, things start to melt very quickly. The arcing generally is not enough to blow the fuse, but is enough to start melting equipment and to possibly start a fire.

The arcing effect would have been apparent when unplugging appliances from the wall without first turning them off. There would have been a significant arc during this process. It may have actually been quite scary to see it!

The AC system does not, in general, suffer from this problem and it is rare to see it. This is due to the AC system having many zero crossings of current and voltage every second. This difference between the two systems would have been noticed by the electrical engineers during the time that both the AC and DC utility systems were in general use, before the decision to standardize on AC was made.

The AC system facilitates the efficient changing of voltages through the use of transformers. Transmitting electricity at high AC voltages was desirable as it uses small cables and saves money. AC motors are much simpler and more reliable.

The DC system would have been emitting large amounts of electromagnetic interference due to the use of brush motors. Brush motors create sparks and increase the risk of fires. It is likely that many people were getting sick around the DC systems due to the dirty electricity on the system.

We see this in some models of cars and motorbikes. Car sickness has a link to the effects of electromagnetic interference on the human body. Most transportation uses DC electrical systems.

The AC system suffers from dirty electricity problems, but was generally cleaner than the DC system until the widespread adoption of electronic systems.

Electric lights do not suffer from flicker on DC systems and the DC system was more desirable for this application.

High powered AC electricity cannot be found in nature and one has to wonder why that is?

"Throughout space there is energy. Is this energy static or kinetic? If static our hopes are in vain; if kinetic - and this we know it is, for certain -then it is a mere question of time when men will succeed in attaching their machinery to the very wheelwork of nature."

Nikola Tesla

50 Hz and 60 Hz

The world has standardized on two forms of AC electricity. Europe has the 50 Hz frequency and America has 60 Hz frequency. There is a mixture of the two systems around the rest of the world.

One has to wonder why there are two frequencies of electrical systems? The frequency was always a trade off between safety and efficiency. The higher the frequency, then the smaller the motors and transformers become. However, increasing frequencies also increase the biological coupling effects and system losses through capacitance and inductance effects.

Believe it or not, the low frequency was chosen to be high enough to prevent the visual perception of flickering electrical lighting products. Electrical lighting was the primary application of the mass market electricity during the early years. Clearly, flickering lighting products would have killed off any consumer markets for the product!

So high enough to prevent visibly flickering lights and low enough to prevent significant coupling effects. It is still unclear as to why two different frequency systems are in use throughout the world and this probably reflects Europe and America being separated in their development of the AC electrical system.

"If there is any one secret of success, it lies in the ability to get the other person's point of view and see things from that person's angle as well as from your own."

Henry Ford

Dirty Electricity

"Dirty Electricity" is the name given to any effects that are on the utility system that are not related to the fundamental system frequency. These effects comprise of:

- Transients.

- Voltage swings.

- Brownouts.

- Surges.

- Lightning.

- Faults.

- Arcing.

- Noise.

- Harmonics.

Transients are generally caused by switching products on or off. Every time a product does this, a transient is generated. It is simply a spike in voltage and current on the system.

Voltage swings occur whenever you turn on or off an appliance on the electrical system. You may see this as the brightness of your lights changing when you use a high powered appliance. What happened was that the voltage changed slightly on the system. This is normal and is simply an effect of the electrical current flowing through the wiring which causes the voltage to change slightly on the electrical system. You may see this frequently in areas with a large amount of solar photovoltaic power generation installed into them. The power feeding in from the solar power systems may cause the voltage to fluctuate, especially on a day with broken clouds.

Brownouts (voltage sag) are caused by high powered items that take much more current than normal to start up. Electrical motors are an example of this. Another example is the utility system switching on a transformer in the area. You may see brownouts whenever these large devices are connected to the electrical system or if the utility is having power supply issues.

Voltage surges are the opposite to brown outs. Large loads being removed from the system may cause the voltage to rise on the system.

Lightning strikes in the area can cause surges and raise the voltage on the grounding system. It is a good reason not to use a swimming pool during a storm.

Faults on the utility system can cause high and low voltages to appear on the system. They will also cause transients.

Arcing of components on the system may cause radio wave emissions to occur. These will travel down the cables and may turn the electrical cables into a radio transmitter.

Noise has many sources to it and comprises of all of the above. The electrical system absorbs energy from its surroundings and there may be frequencies of energy that have got onto it from antenna transmission systems. This is likely to occur in areas closest to the antenna system. Most of the noise is generally low level noise and this can be seen as a wide range of frequencies riding on the utility system voltage sine wave and the combined utility ground (earth) and neutral connections. The main source of noise on the utility system is from harmonics that are generated by equipment that is connected to it and from electronic power generation systems. We will look into this in the next chapter.

"In summary, I believe that there is ample evidence that EMF exposure is associated with increased cancer in humans."

Dr. Sam Milham

Harmonics

Harmonics occur when the current draw from the electrical system is not following the voltage sine wave. Linear loads have a constant impedance and do not create harmonics, and the filament light bulb is a good example of this. The current and voltage waveforms for a filament light bulb is shown in the next picture and you will notice that they both have the smooth sine wave shape. The voltage is the larger sine wave.

When the current draw is not linear (non-sinusoidal), then harmonics occur on the system. Harmonics are higher multiples of frequencies of the electrical system frequency. For 60Hz system, you would get increasing frequencies on the system of 120Hz, 180Hz, 240Hz, 300Hz, 360Hz, 420Hz, and so on. They continue on indefinitely and generally start to diminish their magnitude as the frequencies get higher.

Harmonics are important in understanding the difference between the toxicity of the two different electrical frequency standards of 50Hz and 60Hz. So let us take a look at the 10th, 100th, 1000th and 10,000th harmonic on each system:

50Hz: 500Hz, 5,000Hz, 50,000Hz, 500,000Hz.

60Hz: 600Hz, 6,000Hz, 60,000Hz, 600,000Hz.

Voltage and Current Waveform of a Filament Light Bulb

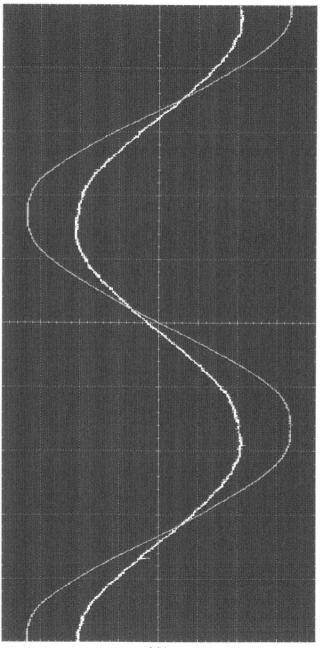

As we can see, the harmonic frequencies are 20% higher on the 60Hz system when compared to the 50Hz system. This matches an observation that I have made that American power engineers appear to be sicker than their British counterparts. It is likely that there is a link to exposure to higher frequency harmonic energy content from the American power system.

Harmonic energy can occur in two ways:

- A non-linear (non-sinusoidal) draw on electrical current that is characteristic of electronic products, street lights, and electronic lighting products.
- A large load on the utility system that deforms the voltage waveform.

You will see the current harmonics long before you see the voltage harmonics.

All electronic products will produce some level of distortion on the current waveform. Some are worse than others. Certain combinations of electronic products on the system may create severe distortions on it. You should be concerned about these distortions as it changes the characteristics of the electrical system emissions into the human environment.

If you are seeing distortion of the voltage sine wave and large amounts of harmonics, you should be really concerned! When troubleshooting a problem like this, you should limit your time in the area, as you may get

sick from excessive electromagnetic interference exposure.

If you look at the waveform in the next image you will see that it is a 60Hz voltage sine wave.

If you look at the same waveform that is on the utility system with an oscilloscope with a fast Fourier transform (FFT) you will see that it looks like the image on the following page. It is normal to see the odd harmonics as they are a feature of all electronic power generation and electronic loads in general. In the image from bottom to top you can see the 60Hz (fundamental), 180Hz (3rd), 300Hz (5th), 420Hz (7th), and 540Hz (9th) harmonics as spikes. The even harmonics generally cancel out on a utility system.

If you have really severe harmonics on the system you will need to start troubleshooting it. Your utility voltage sine wave should never look like the last picture! A waveform like this may make the wiring on the utility system radiate radio waves, magnetic fields, electric fields, and many other forms of electromagnetic radiation!

Utility 60 Hz Voltage Sine Wave

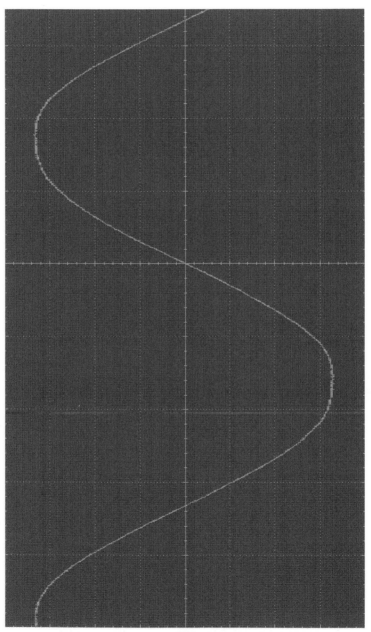

Utility Voltage Harmonics

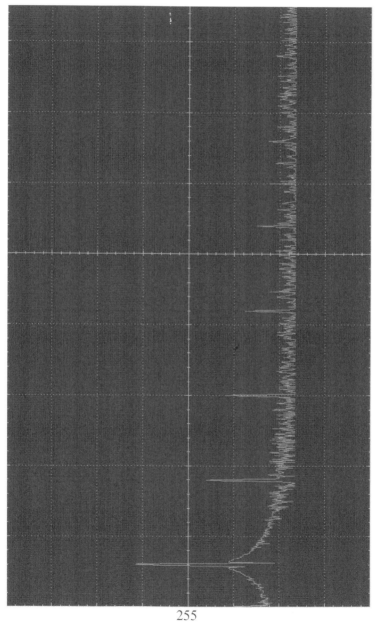

Severe Harmonic Distortion Sine Wave

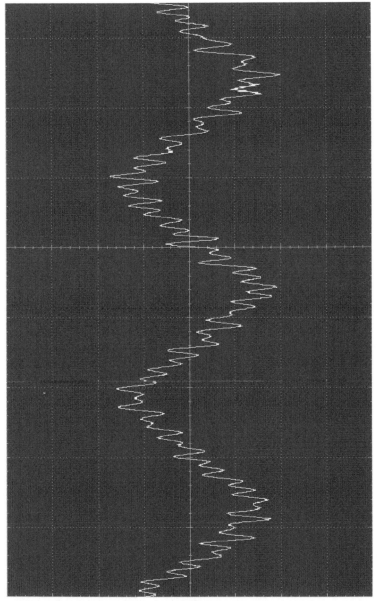

When you put harmonic energy onto an electrical cable, you generally see the following effects occur on cables and equipment:

- Very large electric fields.
- Very large magnetic fields.
- Very large wide band radio wave fields.
- Very large electrostatic fields on high voltage cables.
- Very large ion fields.
- Overloading and overheating.
- Tripping of breakers and blown fuses.
- Exploding fuses.
- Fires.

As you can see, harmonics changes the characteristics of the electrical system considerably and you should avoid using products that generate them.

Individual products that appear to generate low amounts of harmonics may actually start to generate large amounts of harmonics when used in conjunction with other products on your electrical system. The electrical system is always changing with the different times of day, the seasons, and the different loads on the system.

When measuring electrical system harmonics you should do it with a direct connection to the electrical wire. You should avoid using current or voltage transformers to do it as these filter out some of the harmonics. Clamp-on ammeters are relatively useless for accurately reading the system harmonics. You generally will lose all of the high frequency content.

If you cannot use a direct connection to the cable, then you can get an assessment of the harmonics by using a simple AM radio that is tuned to static (no radio station) and using a TriField 100XE meter to read the magnetic and electric field emissions.

I have noticed in the solar photovoltaic industry that usually the best harmonic value is listed on the data sheet and that it does not state if it is the current harmonic or the voltage harmonic that it refers to. To accurately quote electronic inverter harmonic values they should be listed as a low and high range for the current harmonics, and a low and high range for the voltage harmonics as they do vary with the power. A chart showing both values over the power range of the inverter is also useful.

When connecting multiple power generation inverter systems together, this may lead to excessively high harmonics on the electrical system with correspondingly high electromagnetic interference emissions. When assessing inverter systems, the manufacturer should also state the harmonics for the inverter system when there are many utility power generation inverter systems connected to the system. This is called "High Penetration" in the electrical utility industry.

If you want to understand harmonics better, then I can recommend building a harmonic generator. A harmonic generator can easily and cheaply be built using electronic lamp dimmers. The more electronic lamp dimmers and light bulbs that you use, the more extensive the harmonics will be that it generates. You can also install CFL and LED light bulbs that are rated for use with electronic lamp dimmers to increase the harmonic content. Be careful about spending too much time near the harmonic generator, as it may make you sick!

Using a standard AM radio tuned to static (no radio station) and a TriField 100XE meter, you will find some very interesting electromagnetic fields around it. You will be able to see the harmonics by using an oscilloscope with a fast Fourier transform function (FFT). The most extensive harmonics will be found on the neutral current waveform. When using conventional filament light bulbs you will notice that you get very high magnetic fields at low lighting levels and very high electric fields at high lighting levels. The wide band radio wave fields vary with the dimming settings.

The diagram of a harmonic generator test system is shown in the next image and the following picture shows the voltage waveform created by the electronic lamp dimmers.

Harmonic Generator

Live   Neutral

Harmonic Generator Current Waveform.

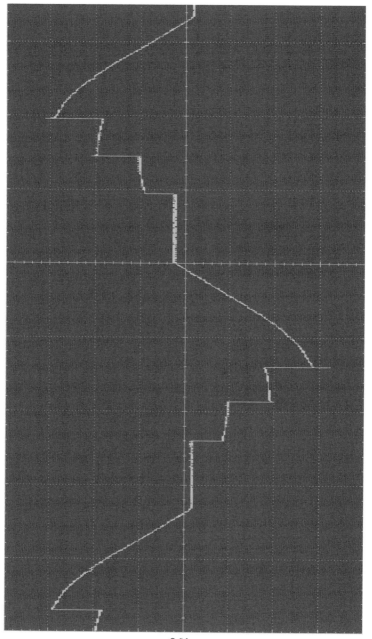

When you test the harmonic generator for magnetic and electric fields, you will find that the peaks for each type of field are in different dimming settings. The peak magnetic field is found by triggering the dimmers before the peak of the voltage waveform and the peak electric field is found by triggering the lamp dimmers after the peak of the voltage waveform.

The following graph shows the current waveform for peak magnetic field overlaid with the peak electric field current waveform.

Peak Electric and Magnetic Field Current Waveforms

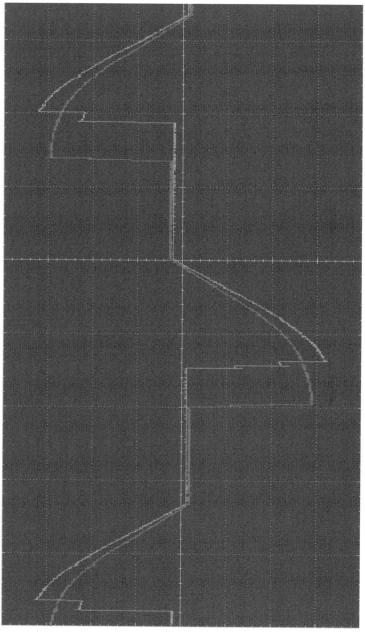

12 volt DC to 120 volt AC inverters used for cars, camping and off grid homes are also good harmonic generators. The cheaper units are called modified sine wave inverters and use square waves to produce the AC power.

I lived in an off grid home for a couple of years and the longer I lived there, the sicker I got! The phone line always buzzed there and this appeared to be an effect of dirty electricity exposure. Off grid homes generally have the poorest power quality and it will vary with the electrical products on the system. I was seeing problems in the two other people that I knew well that lived in off grid homes. One was showing habitual passive aggressiveness and the other was extremely forgetful! Extended dirty electricity exposure may have an intoxication effect that is similar to being on drugs.

The modified sine wave inverter waveform and frequency content can be seen in the next two pictures. The following two pictures show the waveform and frequency content for the more expensive and much better sine wave inverter, note the slightly distorted waveform that causes harmonics to occur. Both types of inverters cause harmonics and the cheaper modified sine wave inverter is horrendous for doing so. I do not recommend extended exposure to these modified sine wave inverter systems, as you may develop some strange health issues.

Modified Sine Wave Inverter Waveform

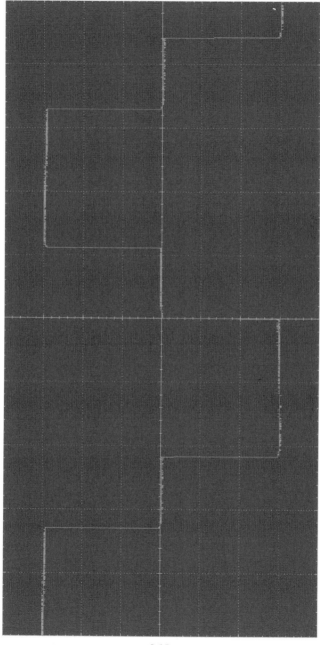

Modified Sine Wave Inverter Frequency Content

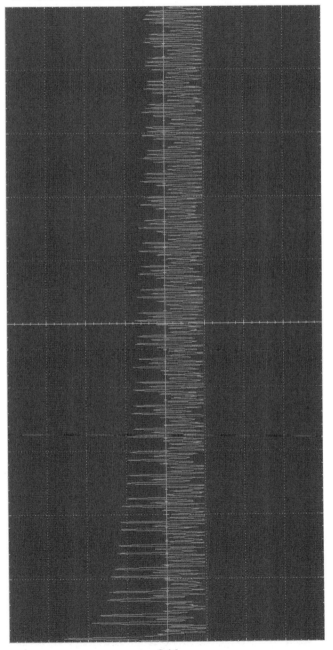

Sine Wave Inverter Waveform

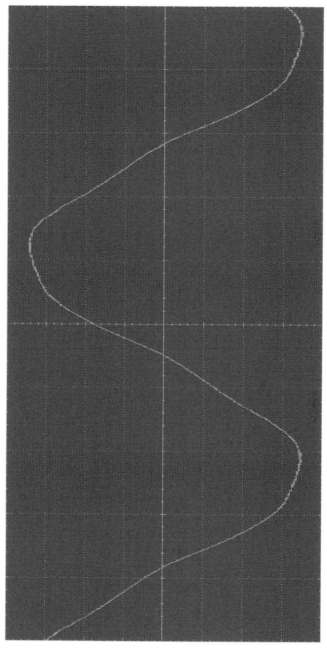

Sine Wave Inverter Frequency Content

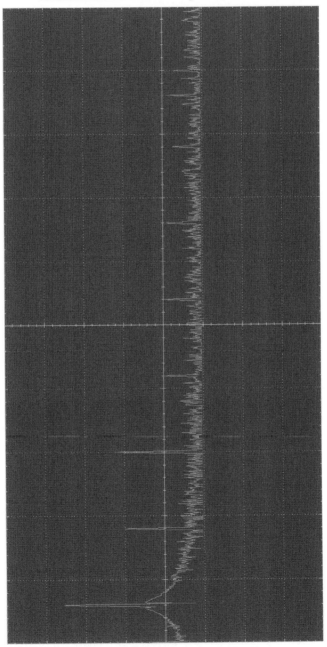

For those with an eye on developing the next hot consumer product, here are a few suggestions:

- Household "Dirty electricity" monitor.

- Household electromagnetic radiation meters.

- Baby room safety scanner for harmful electromagnetic radiation emissions.

- Household "Stray voltage/current/frequency" testers.

To sum up harmonics, I want you to understand that a non-linear current draw is a really bad idea on both AC and DC electrical systems. The more non-linear the current on your electrical system is, then the more toxic your electrical system will become. The cable that supplies the non-linear load may start acting like a radio transmitter! Once there are radio frequencies on the system, then the electrical system may turn everything into a radio transmitter, including the ground that you walk on! Clearly a really bad idea.

"Harmonics are the cancer of the electrical system."

Steven Magee

Direct Electrical Exposure

Direct electrical exposure is the human body coming directly into contact with the electrical system. There appears to be three types of exposure:

- Electrocution.
- Shocks.
- Stray voltage/current/frequency.

We all know that electricity can kill us if we come into contact with the electrical conductors (cables) of the system. The conductors that are energized above earth (ground) potential are called the "Live" conductors and these are the ones that present the risk of electrocution.

Most circuits in the home in the USA are 15 amp circuits. But how much AC current is needed to kill a human? It is a tiny amount of this value. Just 0.02 amp of AC electrical current may kill a human! It is a little lower in the female. A human coming into contact with a live electrical conductor would never blow the fuse.

You need much more DC current than AC current to electrocute a human. For this reason, contact with DC electricity is considered safer than AC.

Most human deaths from electrocution are from these exposures:

270

- Contact with high voltage.
- Contact with voltage where they are unable to let go.
- Burns from electrical current exposure.
- Arc flash.
- Heart attack.

The human body varies in its risk of electrocution. A very dry body needs a much higher amount of voltage to cause electrocution, whereas a wet body needs a much lower level for electrocution. A dry person may be electrocuted on 120 volts AC and a wet person may be electrocuted on just a few volts.

It is for this reason that you see wet areas of homes being protected by ground fault circuit interrupters (GFCI). These sense very low current leakage in the circuit conductors and will trip the circuit if you come into contact with it. If you are working outdoors in the garden with electrical items, you should ensure that your cables are protected by one of these devices.

Most people in the home are electrocuted through not being able to let go of the live conductor that they are in contact with. It causes a grip reaction to occur and paralyzes the human body. Unless you can get yourself off the conductor, you may die from electrical burns or a heart attack. I have experienced this and it is a very strange sensation to lose control of your body. I eventually realized that I could control my legs and kicked my way off the electrical system. I had very deep skin burns on my hands at the entry and exit points of contact with the electrical system.

If you are ever confronted with a person in the process of being electrocuted, do not go near them or touch them. Find the circuit breaker and turn it off. If you do not know where it is, find a dry wooden pole and push them off the electrical system. If they are in a wet area, you should not enter the area. If you do not know where the circuit breaker is located and it is not accessible, you should consider shorting the circuit to trip the breaker. Do not short high powered circuits as you may get arc flash issues. You will need to act quickly to save the persons life, but do not act in a way that could endanger your own life. If you cannot get them off the electrical system, call the emergency services. A person who has had a severe shock should be sent to the hospital for evaluation, as they may have internal damage that may show up later.

Arc flash is not electrocution, but it can kill a person. It happens around high energy equipment failures and it is a radiation exposure. The radiation emitted by arcing electricity irradiates the human body, causing extensive radiation burns. It is the burns that kill the person. This is a particular problem in the utility industry.

Electrical welders have a similar problem to arc flash. In welders, it generally causes a sunburn reaction, as the arc is not high powered. "Arc Eye"(Photokeratitis) is a condition associated with welders and is the reason why you see them using face shields. You should never watch a welder working, otherwise you may develop arc eye. Welders are a group of people who get extensive exposure to stray voltage/current/frequency and electromagnetic radiation emissions.

Shocks are caused by coming into contact with electrical currents that are high enough to be sensed by the human body but are low enough not to kill it. So how much current is needed to sense electricity in the human? Dr. William B. Kouwenhoven, a professor of electrical engineering at John Hopkins university, found that it is about 0.003 amp of AC current. 0.006 amp AC causes a painful shock in the female and 0.009 amp AC is needed for pain in the male. It is important to note that the female is more vulnerable than the male to electrical exposures.

DC shocks can be far worse than AC shocks. One of the worst electrical shocks that I have ever had was from a 330 volt DC circuit. It was so bad that I had a headache for a week afterwords! The difference between AC and DC is noticeable when you are in contact with it. The AC shock sends pulses of electricity through the human body that can be felt. The DC shock is just continuous.

Stray voltage/current/frequency is the most serious form of exposure. Electrocution kills very few people per year. Stray voltage/current/frequency exposure is suspected to be making people sick in the millions!

It is quite possible that tens of thousands of deaths per year in the USA have stray voltage/current/frequency at their root cause. The problem with stray voltage/current/frequency exposure is that the symptoms vary with the voltage, current and frequencies of the electricity that the person is exposed to. No two people will have the same exposures. Around stray voltage/current/frequency the persons exposure will vary according to their lifestyle. Things that will increase stray voltage/current/frequency exposure are:

- Copper plumbing.

- Cast iron drains.

- Swimming.

- Hot tub.

- Location of grounding rods.

- Conductive tiled floors.

- Conductive concrete floors.

- Conductive counters.

- Conductive brick home.

- Conductive metal home.

- Conductive shoes.

- Walking a dog.

- Sitting or laying on conductive flooring.

- Their career.

- Their electrical utility company.

- Their electrical and electronic products.

- Dirty electricity.

- The presence of an alternate energy system in the area.

As you can see, there are a lot of variables that feed into your exposure to stray voltage/current/frequency. You

should assume that wherever electricity is installed, that there is a risk of stray voltage/current/frequency exposure. You will not be able to feel it, you will just notice that your health is mysteriously deteriorating.

Stray voltage/current/frequency is poorly understood and is one of the biggest threats to long term human health around electrical systems.

"Someone confronted with an electrocution, for example, usually stands there helplessly."

Susanne Woelk

Lightning

Lightning is nature's electricity. Our knowledge of electricity was developed from it. Wikipedia states:

Lightning is an atmospheric electrical discharge (spark) accompanied by thunder, usually associated and produced by cumulonimbus clouds, but also occurring during volcanic eruptions or in dust storms. From this discharge of atmospheric electricity, a leader of a bolt of lightning can travel at speeds of 220,000 km/h (140,000 mph), and can reach temperatures approaching 30,000 °C (54,000 °F), hot enough to fuse silica sand into glass channels known as fulgurites, which are normally hollow and can extend as much as several meters into the ground. There are some 16 million lightning storms in the world every year. Lightning causes ionization in the air through which it travels, leading to the formation of nitric oxide and ultimately, nitric acid, of benefit to plant life below.

Lightning is high voltage, high current DC electricity and can have positive or negative polarity. When a lightning strike occurs it generates an electromagnetic field. This can be heard on a standard AM radio that is tuned into static (no radio station). If there is a lot of lightning in the area then you will hear a lot of noise on the AM radio.

The lightning strike occurs when the electrical breakdown of air is reached, typically at one million volts per meter. When the lightning passes through the air it heats it to three times hotter than the surface of the Sun! The strongest electromagnetic radiation produced appears to be below 300,000 Hertz. This is called the low frequency (LF) and very low frequency (VLF) ranges. Lightning also has a significant amount of energy in the high frequency range (HF) up to 30,000,000Hz.

There are two wave types associated with lightning. The ground wave is the direct line of sight electromagnetic radiation from the storm. The sky wave is the reflected electromagnetic radiation from the ionosphere part of the atmosphere.

Lightning produces wide band radio waves by pulsing the DC current. These pulsing DC currents cause a wide range of frequencies to be generated. It can be compared to dirty electricity. One of the reasons that dirty electricity is so harmful to the human is that it is not seasonal, it is continually in the modern human environment. The human is designed to only have short exposures annually to lightning storms.

When listening to the lightning storms in your area on a standard AM radio, you will hear a sound like bacon frying and this is the electromagnetic energy that the storm is generating. Plants react to this energy and may show vigorous growth during lightning seasons.

It is quite possible that crime is tied to the electromagnetic emissions from lightning. The high amount of electromagnetic energy in the area may affect human mental health and trigger a crime spree. This may be especially the case in areas that are prone to large amounts of lightning like Florida, USA.

For human health purposes, you may want to avoid living in areas that are prone to high levels of lightning. Certain parts of Florida may actually have too much lightning in them for it to be considered safe for humans to inhabit long term. Too much lightning may bring about the symptoms of radio wave sickness and electromagnetic hypersensitivity. Fatigue is the top reported symptom and you may see it appear during periods of seasonal lightning storms and disappear outside of these times of year. If you live in a high lightning area and are seeing seasonal fatigue occurring, you should consider moving away from the area.

There are no doubts that electromagnetic radiation exposure can trigger the human mating cycle and it is quite possible that birth rates may be tied to lightning!

Lightning strike rates increase in areas that the man-made structures exceed the height of trees. The higher the structure is, the greater the increase in lightning strikes in the area. It increases by approximately the square of the height of the structure. Lightning travels relatively slowly through the air but increases to the speed of light when it travels through a metal conductor to the ground below. This causes increased radiation emissions from the lightning strike which may affect people in the surrounding area.

Downtown areas will be more prone to lightning due to their tall buildings and people who live near to these areas may actually find that there are too many lightning strikes taking place at close proximity to them. They may actually get overloaded on electromagnetic exposure from the lightning strikes! You should avoid living in areas that have tall structures that short circuit the atmospheric layers as the long term health problems are currently unknown.

Lightning rods on tall structures short circuit the atmospheric layers. This can be seen when studying lightning strikes. The lightning will come down through the atmosphere as normal, but when it hits the short circuited atmospheric layer it will travel horizontally to the lightning rod where it discharges down the lightning conductor to the ground. As it does so, it fills that area with electromagnetic radiation emissions that are distinctly different from what the storm naturally produces. This is shown in the next diagram.

Lightning & Short Circuited Atmospheric Layers

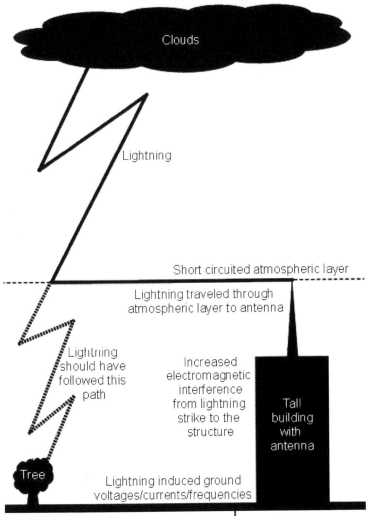

Lightning will tend to hit the tallest structure in the area. Trees, towers and power lines all have the same probability of being hit if they are at the same height. However, the frequency emissions appear to be different between the man-made objects and those of nature.

Lightning is well known for its ability to damage electrical and electronic products. A close lightning strike raises the voltage on the utility electrical system and can destroy electrical and electronic products. Another effect of nearby lighting strikes is that they produce significant levels of radio frequencies. These will be induced into anything that is acting as an antenna system and may create damage to the system. Some solar photovoltaic power systems are known to be affected by this, as the solar modules and electrical wiring create a large antenna system.

Airplane pilots are at risk of lightning exposure and may get intoxicated from it when flying through an electrical storm. The electrical activity will envelop the airplane in St. Elmo's Fire and create very high electromagnetic radiation levels inside the airplane. The pilots may display poor brain functioning, aggression, poor senses, human senses may be reporting information that is not true, human actions may not reflect thoughts, and confusion. This appears to be what happened in the Air France flight 447 crash.

The problem with subjecting the human to man-made electromagnetic interference fields is that the human exposure to EMI is seasonal. Subjecting the human to daily EMI from electrical, electronic and wireless products is comparable to constantly sitting in the middle of a high intensity lighting storm! Clearly an unnatural activity.

Accompanying lightning is a shock wave. This is what we hear as thunder. It is a supersonic wave that is created by the rapid expansion of the heated air. The shock wave is likely to have an affect on the human as well. Supersonic shock waves are associated with heart problems.

One of the problems with climate change, global warming and global air pollution is that it may change the frequency and intensity of electrical storm activity. Too much lightning activity may cause excessive mating, aggression, fatigue, illness and disease to occur. Too little may turn off the animal and plant breeding cycles.

We know that static ceases to occur at above 30% relative humidity. As the Earth's atmosphere heats up, the humidity will fall and may turn on major static electrical activity in the atmosphere. The falling humidity levels may also turn off the lightning storms! With no clouds, there will be no electrical storms.

"Electricity is really just organized lightning."
George Carlin

Static

Static is an electrical charge that forms on dissimilar materials and objects due to the differences of movement between them.

When an object is charged up with static, the fibers repel from each other. This also happens to the human and the body hair will stand up. Synthetic materials generate this effect when in contact with the human body. You need to be careful with clothes that generate static, as they may have you walking around in a static generated electromagnetic field! You can hear this effect with an AM radio tuned to static (no radio station). Every time you see a spark, you will hear it on the radio.

High humidity kills static. This is why sometimes you may see it and other times not. If the clothes are humid you will not see the effect. Having plants inside your home humidifies your home and helps to prevent static from occurring.

In the past people used to wear leather soled shoes and these were good for keeping the person electrically grounded to the side walk. They provide a discharge path for the static. Today, you should be wearing insulated shoes, due to the presence of electrified ground near to electrical grounding systems. With insulated shoes, you should ensure that you are wearing natural clothing in order not to generate the static. Insulated shoes that generate static should be avoided, as they may make you sick!

It is quite possible that some people's illnesses are tied to the static discharges that are occurring in their environment. The radio wave fields that it generates may cause electromagnetic hypersensitivity to occur and this is why it is important to wear natural clothing.

Static is generally very high voltage and very low current. We are lucky that the current is low, otherwise we would all be dying from electrocution!

"We tested his clothes with a static electricity field meter and measured a current of 40,000 volts, which is one step shy of spontaneous combustion, where his clothes would have self-ignited."

Henry Barton

Direct Current (DC)

Most people associate direct current (DC) with batteries. It has a constant voltage that does not change over time. In nature you find DC electricity in areas such as:

- Swamps.

- Bogs.

- Marshes.

- Moors.

- The tree canopy.

- The atmosphere.

Atmospheric energy has direct current in it and it has a voltage gradient that is negative for the first couple of miles above the ground and that then changes to positive polarity as you go higher into the atmosphere. Close to the ground the voltage increase is between 1 to 19 volts per foot. Flying kites with conductive strings will expose you to this atmospheric voltage, as will helium balloons with long conductive strings. Higher up in the atmosphere, the voltage increases by approximately 30 volts per foot.

All living organisms that stand tall on the ground are subjected to this DC voltage and this is evidenced in the following pictures.

The Dieffenbachia grows well regardless of if the voltage is positive or negative 1.5 volts on its stem relative to the roots. It indicates that the atmospheric DC voltage polarity may reverse in nature over time. I can only get the Dieffenbachia to grow normally at my home by using a 1.5 volt battery which indicates that the atmospheric DC voltage in my area has changed, which is very concerning!

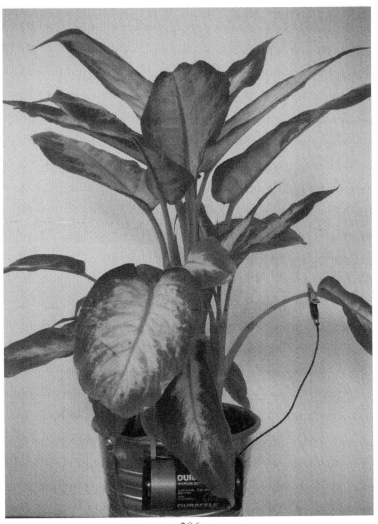

If the DC voltage gets too high, then the Dieffenbachia plant starts to show stress. 9 volts positive polarity on the stem appears to cause growth defects (shown) and seems more harmful than 9 volts negative stem polarity that seems to stunt growth and corrodes the metal alligator clip.

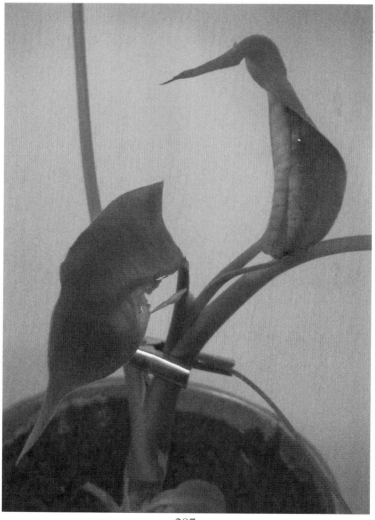

My plants are grown in high radiation fields that appear to come from radio frequency transmitting utility meters and three cell phone towers that are between 600-700 meters from my home. The Dieffenbachia's all deform at my home regardless of where they are grown at on my property. The only ones that grow normally have 1.5 DC volts on them! As we can see in the plants, we can restore the normal growth patterns by applying a DC voltage to them. The voltage has to be kept to the correct level, otherwise stresses will show up if too high or too low. Applying a DC voltage between the soles of the feet of the human and the upper body may have applications in the field of human health. This is shown in the next diagram.

I am currently experimenting with putting the human mind and body into a DC electric field during sleep. I have a large sheet of conductive aluminum foil attached to the 10' high ceiling above the bed and a large sheet of conductive aluminum foil on the floor under the bed to effect this. The upper sheet is connected to the negative terminal of a battery and the lower sheet is connected to the positive terminal. This can be seen in the following photograph.

The upper sheet is akin to the tree canopy which is known to have a DC voltage on it. A company called Voltree Power (www.voltreepower.com) is developing the use of tree voltage to power electronic systems and has extensively researched the DC voltage of trees.

The feet are connected together through being in contact with the conductive ground and are earthed (grounded). The mind and body are walking around in a DC voltage field. That DC voltage will energize the mind and body and the lack of it may make the human sick.

Human Electrical Model

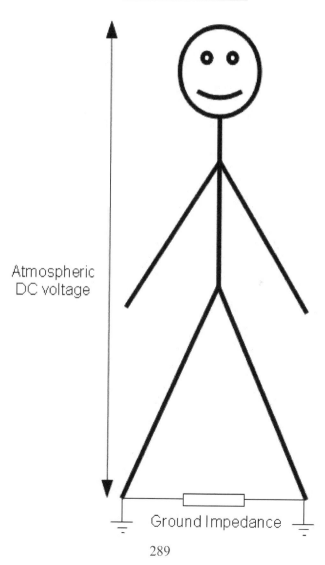

Atmospheric DC voltage

Ground Impedance

The upper and lower sheets of aluminum foil are the same size as the bed. The DC voltage on the conductive sheets will set up a DC voltage field between them with a small flow of electrons that should pass through the human sleeping in the bed. This is currently an unproven experimental health technique that may have unknown side effects. I call this technique: "Electromagnetic Sandwich"

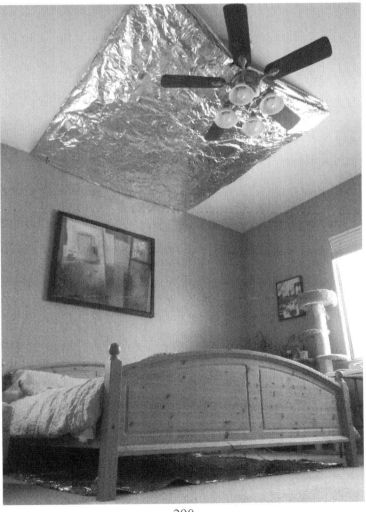

I started testing the electromagnetic sandwich with a 9 volt battery which should give approximately 2 volts of a negative atmospheric voltage exposure to my mind and body during sleep. The atmospheric voltage gradient between the floor sheet and the ceiling negative sheet is 0.9 volt DC per foot. I could definitely feel the difference when I was sleeping and headaches and muscle weakness showed up after about a week of testing. I changed the battery to 1.5 volt DC and found that this was much more agreeable to human health and the health problems cleared up. 1.5 volts DC appears to be more comparable to what you find on the tree canopy. I may adjust the DC voltage later, depending on what I find with long term testing.

It is interesting that the human health difference in the DC voltage exposures matches what I saw in the Dieffenbachia plants. Exposure to a very low DC voltage that is comparable a single DC battery cell appears healthy for biological systems and 9 volts DC stresses them.

My initial assessment of the electromagnetic sandwich health technique is that the occasional daytime fatigue that I was experiencing has been significantly reduced. I find this very concerning, as it indicates that a DC atmospheric voltage is missing at my home that is required for both good plant health and good human health. It appears that people who suffer from electromagnetic hypersensitivity may be reacting to this loss of atmospheric DC voltage. They appear to be the electromagnetic radiation equivalent of the "Coalminers canary" and it is very foolish to ignore the health symptoms that these many people are reporting. They are very clearly reacting to unnatural man-made electromagnetic radiation conditions.

I have further developed the electromagnetic sandwich technique for daytime use. It is easily implemented using an anti-static wrist strap and an anti-static mat. This is shown in the next picture. For those of you on the go, you can wear an anti-static heel strap and an anti-static wrist strap and just put the 1.5 volt DC battery in your pocket. Keep the cables as short as possible and it is preferable to use straight cables as opposed to the coiled cables shown in the picture. Long cables and cable coils act as antenna systems and will put strange frequencies onto the DC voltage that may lead to electromagnetic hypersensitivity.

These health techniques are experimental and have unknown side effects at the time of writing. The DC voltages may require adjusting to higher or lower levels and will be person dependent due to the impedance of the fat to muscle ratio. They may need to only be applied for short periods rather than continuous use. This is a developing area of research that is very new and there are a lot of unknowns currently.

If you choose to implement them, you should be under qualified and competent medical supervision and discontinue the techniques if adverse health symptoms show up. You would be assuming any and all risks using these health techniques.

During the daytime I am now experimenting with wearing an anti-static strap on my wrist that is connected to the negative terminal of a 1.5 volt DC battery. The positive terminal is connected to an anti-static mat that my bare feet rest on. This creates a DC voltage gradient across my body that is similar to what nature does. Both the mat and the wrist strap have 1,000,000 ohm resistors built into them.

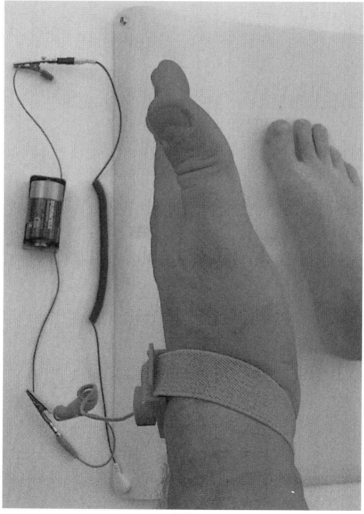

High powered DC batteries are used for industrial applications and are commonly found in vehicles and battery powered systems. I have found fields around these batteries, so you should be careful with exposure to them. People that I have met who work full time with high powered batteries tend to have strange personalities and is likely due to daily exposure to them.

Batteries tend to be low voltage and each battery cell is about 1 to 2 volts, depending on the technology used. Higher voltage batteries are simply a collection of many battery cells connected together in series. You need to be careful with such high voltage batteries and a DC shock can be more severe than an AC shock. Both can kill you.

"We cannot hope to either understand or to manage the carbon in the atmosphere unless we understand and manage the trees and the soil too."

Freeman Dyson

Faraday Cages & Screening

Faraday cages have been around for hundreds of years. First reports of them were by Benjamin Franklin and Micheal Faraday documented the use of these cages for protection from electricity sources. They have been known as Faraday cages ever since.

David Blaine recently demonstrated the phenomenon in his October 2012 "Electrified" show. Standing for three days and three nights surrounded by numerous million volt Tesla coils, he was repeatedly hit by high voltage sparks. He was wearing a metal "Faraday cage" suit and an open wire frame helmet. He did appear to get shocked during the show and he was reporting that his skin was tingling during practice. It was clear that the suit was not fully protective of the energies that he was exposed to.

I did try and contact David Blaine to get feedback on the health symptoms that showed up before, during and after the show, but no reply was ever received. I have never seen a public statement issued by him regarding this subject either. I am curious to know what health symptoms showed up and if there were any lasting effects from the exposures that he received from the "Electrified" show. If you know what happened, I would like to hear from you.

David Blaine demonstrated one of the myths surrounding Faraday cages and that is if you are inside a Faraday cage, that you are fully protected from the energies that are outside of it. This is not true. Faraday cages are simply attenuators for energy transmission through the surrounding atmosphere. They reduce some energies more than others. The energy reduction effect is frequency dependent and a Faraday cage may significantly reduce some frequencies and may only slightly reduce others. Many energies will pass into the Faraday cage, generally with attenuation.

Tesla coil performers generally report a feeling of euphoria and it probably comes from the intense flashes of light, the electromagnetic exposures and the gasses that they breath during the show. The Telsa coil performer should be wearing ultraviolet blocking glasses during the show due to the ultraviolet emissions from the sparks. Muscle soreness may be reported afterwords. The electromagnetic exposures for a Tesla coil performer are increased if they are in contact with the Faraday cage. High frequency electromagnetic exposure is known for its effects on the brain and is linked to increased rates of brain tumors. Tesla coil performers should be aware of the symptoms of electromagnetic hypersensitivity in case they start to develop it. The audience is also at risk of developing some of the above problems.

Faraday cages are commonly grounded to discharge the energy. While energy discharge is needed around high powered equipment, we know today that sometimes it is actually healthier to leave the Faraday cage ungrounded. It is one of the myths that is around that they only function effectively against high frequency radiation sources when they are grounded. I have done extensive testing of Faraday cages around AM and FM radio receivers and 2.4 gigahertz Wi-Fi transmitters and have found no noticeable performance gain in the electromagnetic shielding properties of these Faraday cages when grounded. It is quite the opposite. If you connect a Faraday cage into a source of stray voltage/frequency/current, then you may turn it into a transmitter!

Regarding electromagnetic hypersensitivity, people have been using the principles of Faraday cages to protect themselves from radio frequency sources. They have noticed that grounding them sometimes increases their symptoms and they use their Faraday cages ungrounded.

Plants do not grow correctly inside Faraday cages and may show abnormal branching, leaf size, stalky growth patterns and unusual growth rates. Dr. John Nash Ott noted the natural cycles were interrupted in plants that he took to the bottom of a coal mine. This is in line with work that has been done in the past that shows that when the human is disconnected from surface radiation effects that the biological cycles become affected. The experts on this subject are the manned Space programs. Spaceships and space stations are nothing more than Faraday cages that are in extremely unnatural environments. Astronauts show many health problems when living in Space and typically only spend several months there. I find it very concerning that people who are suffering from electromagnetic hypersensitivity are now resorting to living in Faraday cages! This may cause radiation deficiency conditions in the long term.

The growth effects of a Dieffenbachia plant that was grown in an ungrounded aluminum window mesh Faraday cage is shown in the next photograph.

This Dieffenbachia has spent eleven months living inside an ungrounded Faraday cage. It is showing extensive growth problems that include very small leaves, loss of patterning and abnormal branching structure.

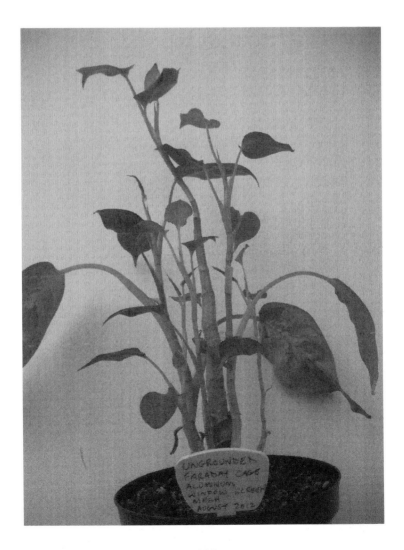

Similar to the Faraday cage is electromagnetic shielding. People who have electromagnetic hypersensitivity are known to install shielding where there are sources of radio frequencies. They have noticed that grounding these electromagnetic shields sometimes makes their symptoms worse and they will disconnect the ground for improved health. The shield becomes a transmitter of radio frequencies when connected to dirty electrical grounding systems. It is also well documented in the field of antenna systems that grounding antennas increases the radio frequency content and energy on them.

Electromagnetic shielding fabric is sold and many people with electromagnetic hypersensitivity use it. It tends to have conductive threads woven into it. Some people have noticed that when it is in contact with their skin, it can make them sicker. If they have the shielding fabric with an air gap between it and their skin, then they get the benefits of reduced radio frequency exposure. It appears that these shielding fabrics can act as antenna systems and couple the radio frequencies on them into the human when they are in contact with it.

Installing shielding onto a single wall can create an electromagnetic reflector. Electromagnetic waves that hit it at the correct angle may cause what is known as an interference pattern to occur near to it. Interference causes zones of much higher levels of radiation to occur. Many people are reporting that they install shielding and it makes them sick. It is likely that a radio frequency interference pattern is set up in the shielded room.

There is a difference between the shielding materials in general use for radio frequency protection and they are listed in the order of my recommendation:

1. Radio frequency (RF) absorbing paint: This is the most expensive shielding material and is the preference to use due to it absorbing the radio frequency signal rather than reflecting it. However, it is very difficult to remove later.

2. Aluminum foil: This has the best radio frequency signal blocking properties but is reflective to them and may create interference patterns.

3. Aluminum window screening mesh: This is effective at blocking most radio frequency signals, but will let through some very high frequencies. It is reflective to radio frequencies and may create interference patterns.

4. Space blankets (Mylar film): The quality of space blankets varies and it tends to be the worst performing electromagnetic shield. It is available in large sheets and many people have used it successfully to reduce radio frequency levels. It is reflective to radio frequencies and may create interference patterns.

It is preferable to have shields that have a distorted surface to them. This is so that they will reflect the radio frequency signal from them as a scattered signal. This will reduce the chances of setting up high powered interference patterns near to them. If using space blankets or aluminum foil, simply crumple it up before installing it. Loosely install it so that the surface stays distorted.

Regarding mesh shields, these typically perform better the smaller the holes are within the mesh. Mesh shields are regarded as needing the holes to be smaller than 1/10 of a wavelength of the highest frequency that you are shielding from.

When connecting your electromagnetic shield to ground, then you should make your ground cable to be exactly a multiple of half the wavelength that you are trying to shield against. Cable impedance to high frequencies is high at quarter wavelengths and low at half wavelengths. It is desirable to have low impedance grounding with shielding.

Some people who have electromagnetic hypersensitivity sleep inside of conductive bed canopies that look similar to mosquito nets. The bed canopy shielding has mixed reports and it works for some and not for others. The technique may be modified by the insertion of an appropriate voltage battery and resistor between the non-electrified ground rod and the bed canopy. The resistor should be sized to keep the current limited to one milliamp for safety. For a 1.5 volt battery, you would use a 1,500 ohm resistor in series with it. So the bed canopy would have a low level DC voltage on it relative to the ground below.

You need to be careful with creating Faraday cages and electromagnetic shielding for human health purposes. You may create electromagnetic deficiencies in the human that are similar to what is observed in the astronauts on the International Space Station. If you choose to use electromagnetic shielding techniques, you should be monitoring your long term health and discontinue the techniques if health issues start to show up.

People are inadvertently living in excessively electromagnetically shielded homes and this may occur from the use of radiant foil barriers, the use of insulation that has electromagnetic shielding properties, metal roofs, metal siding, windows that have electromagnetic shielding properties, and so on.

"The Hum" is a steady droning sound that can only be heard by a small group of people and they report headaches, nausea, dizziness, nosebleeds and sleep disturbances. These match closely to the conditions reported for electromagnetic hypersensitivity. Someone contacted me about "The Hum" and they said it started when they installed aluminum foil radiant barrier attic insulation in their home and it cleared up when they moved home. They essentially had a lot of ungrounded aluminum foil in their attic in close proximity to their electrical cables for the lighting circuits! They had created a very unnatural electromagnetic radiation environment which they appeared to be reacting to.

Electromagnetic shielding is a tricky subject and you should not be engaging in the practice unless you understand the biological consequences. You should be using an RF meter to enable you to confirm effective shielding from a known biologically harmful source. The only area of my home that has shielding in it is the garage where the transmitting utility meters are located.

"Every great advance in science has issued from a new audacity of imagination."

John Dewey

Biological Coupling

There are many ways that the human may be affected by exposure to electrical energy. Most people associate shocks and electrocution as the way electricity harms people. The truth is, this is just a small fraction of the overall harm that is being done to the human. The human is constantly coming into contact with electricity through:

- Electromagnetic field exposure.
- Stray voltage/current/frequency from electrical grounding systems.

There is a more serious effect than electrocution and shocks that may be occurring in various parts of the body. Loops are present throughout the human body and some are obvious and others are more discrete. Some of the places that you will find loops in the human body are:

- Inner Ear.
- Eye pupil.
- Eye orbit.
- Nostril.
- Spinal column.
- Collar bone.
- Circular bone surrounding marrow.
- Esophagus.

- Lungs.

- Heart.

- Rib cage.

- Intestines.

- Kidneys.

- Ovaries and fallopian tubes.

- Hips.

- Blood cells.

- Arteries, veins, and capillaries.

Why are loops a concern? Because they may couple into the electrical fields by a process called "induction". Induction may cause electrical currents to flow within the loops when in the presence of electromagnetic fields. Flowing currents through these loops may cause illness or disease to occur. The currents may cause localized heating, electric and magnetic fields.

The red blood cells are known to stick together when in electromagnetic fields. Exposure to sunlight frees them. It is called a Rouleaux formation in the medical field.

Man-made loops may be present on the human body and we see these in various locations:

- Eye wear.

- Earrings.

- Necklace.

- Rings.

- Bangles.

- Bracelets.

- Watches.

You should also be wary of any kind of metal on the human body. In particular, the curved metal wire in under-wired bra's has already been identified as acting like a reflector for focusing radio and microwaves into the breast tissue. Metal zippers can have similar effects.

You should avoid letting the medical profession install metal into your body like metal fillings, metal bridges and metal implants. Galvanic effects may occur between different metals on and inside the body. The body acts as an electrolyte and creates ion flows between the metals.

Any metal in electromagnetic fields may have voltages and frequencies induced into it. An under wire that I tested in the field of a 32 inch cathode ray tube TV had a very distorted AC voltage waveform on it and a wide range of frequencies. These are different between the under wires and the two under wires appear to create an electrical circuit through the human body.

It is interesting to note that during research into how electric shocks affect humans, it was noted that the female body is more sensitive than the male. This is a concern as women tend to wear far more metal on their bodies than men which increases their electromagnetic exposures.

In the UK, women generally have more cancer than men and that may be coming from exposure to kitchen and laundry appliances. Extended time in these areas of the home may increase a persons risk of illness and disease, as these appliances generally have large electromagnetic fields around them. Electronically controlled appliances tend to be worse than basic appliances.

A similar effect to the under-wired bra may occur in the astronomical field, but on a much larger scale. Metal observatory domes may act as reflectors that focus radio and microwaves. Any curved metal structure may exhibit this focusing effect. You should not use transmitting devices in such environments.

Any metal structure may be able to cause radio and microwave reflections to occur and you should be wary of using products that create electromagnetic waves in locations such as these. The pictures on the following pages demonstrate these effects.

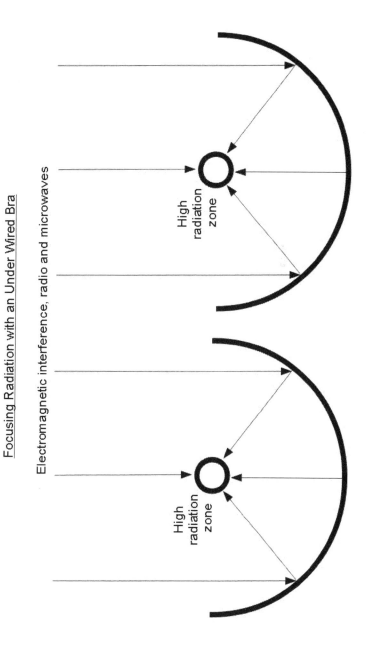

Focusing Radiation with an Under Wired Bra

Electromagnetic interference, radio and microwaves

High radiation zone

High radiation zone

The highly distorted 60 Hz AC waveform between the under wires in the field of the 32 inch cathode ray tube TV

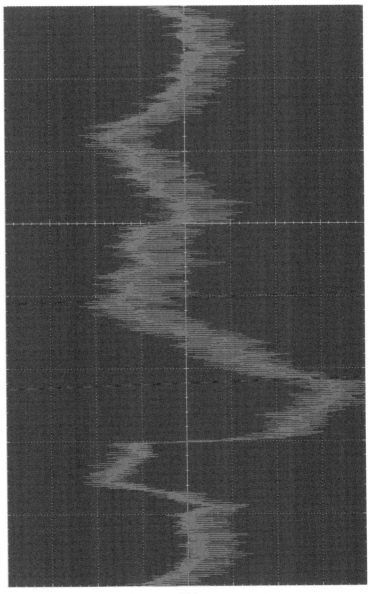

The metal under wired bra can have a wide range of
frequencies on it when in electromagnetic fields. The
repeating spikes are the harmonics.

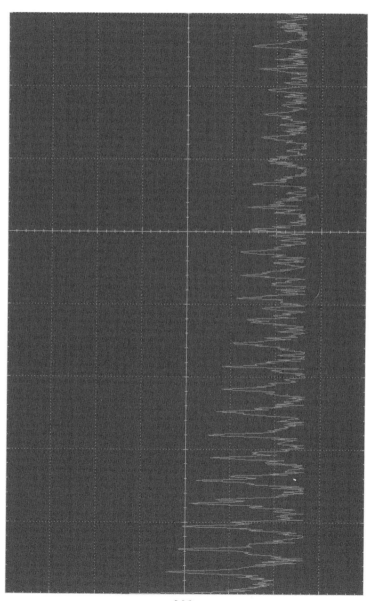

Metal Dome Radiation Reflections

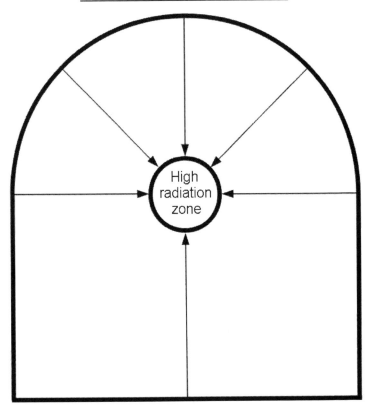

Any transmitting device in the center of the dome will create a high radiation area from the reflected waves

The human nervous system never connects in a loop and this is probably to prevent electrical induction effects from occurring in it. Instead the nerves are balanced between the left and right side of the human body, feeding out radially from the spinal cord to the various bodily systems that they connect to.

One of the problems of these man-made electromagnetic fields is that they are not uniform. They rapidly fall off with distance from the source. This means that part of the human body may be in a high radiation field and part of it may be in a low radiation field. It may create currents that flow around the body between the low and high radiation exposure areas. It is an undesirable effect.

The rise of Female Hysteria in the 1800's when the ladies were wearing steel hoop skirts and steel crinolines was followed with the development of the vibrator. Female Hysteria caused the female mating cycle to be triggered and created a demand for genital stimulation devices. Unfortunately, the vibrator is a sex product that really should be avoided due to the electromagnetic fields that they may emit. This is especially concerning for internal vibrators, as the human body has no natural protection from internally generated electromagnetic fields. Vibrators are known to be addictive and this may be related to the electromagnetic interference from it repeatedly triggering the mating cycle and reinforcing the desire to use it.

Wearing shoes and clothing that create static is really undesirable. Static creates radio waves and may induce electromagnetic hypersensitivity into you. You should pay attention to the shoes and clothes that your children wear and if you find that they are generating static discharges, then you should identify the item that is generating the static and discard it.

High powered alternating current electricity does not occur in nature and it is wise to exercise caution around it. There must be a reason why nature does not use it and it would be foolish to ignore this. All high powered electricity in nature is direct current (DC). The electric eel is a good example of this and it can generate a voltage of approximately 500 volts to stun its prey. Thunderstorms also produce large DC voltages of millions of volts and we see this as lightning. It appears that Edison was right to promote the use of DC electricity in the famous "War of the Currents" that he had with Tesla's AC system.

Radio waves do occur in nature and these generally are seasonal with the arrival of lighting storms. It appears that the electromagnetic radiation that nature produces is a stimulant to the human mind and body for fertility and also sexual desire. Given that humans have now filled their environments with radio waves all year round, it should come as no surprise that we have seen unprecedented growth in human population over the last century. The human body may now be extremely fertile all year with a constant desire to mate, as opposed to the fertility and mating cycles following the seasons in the past. I call this:

Electromagnetic Population Growth

Fortunately, the human body does appear to have an electrical noise reduction system built into its nervous system. The nervous system is widely acknowledged to be driven by electrical impulses, so this is not a surprise. The left part of the brain controls the right side of the body and the right part of the brain controls the left side of the body. This twist that occurs appears to be an electrical noise reduction technique that enables the body to function in high EMI environments. This is shown on the following page.

Human Body Electromagnetic Field Cancellation

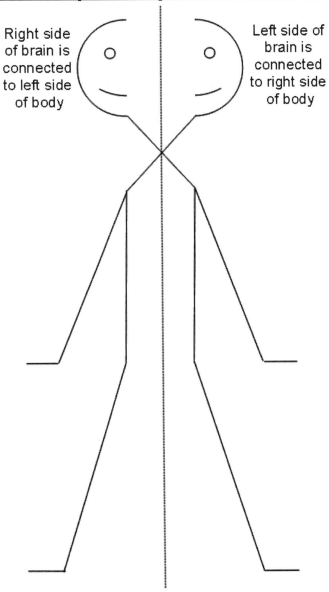

Right side of brain is connected to left side of body

Left side of brain is connected to right side of body

The nervous system uses electrical noise reduction techniques

The back and forth structures of the brain and intestines may also be an electrical noise canceling technique. The arteries and veins generally run next to each other and this is another electrical noise reduction effect. DNA double helix spirals may be acting as Faraday cages to electromagnetically screen the DNA code. Electrical noise reduction techniques are present throughout the body.

There are certain parts of the body that may act like antennas and these may be:

- Brain.
- Brain near temples.
- Eyes.
- Body.
- Spinal cord.
- Intestines.
- Arms.
- Legs.
- Feet.
- Digits.
- Hair.
- Testicles.
- Penis.
- Breasts.
- G-Spot.

Regarding the brain and intestines, they may also be functioning as fractal antennas and extracting energy and radiating energy. The human mating and fertility cycle is triggered by exposure to lightning storms and it is likely that all of the above areas are involved in the process.

It is well known that when the human is placed into an unnatural electromagnetic environment that this affects the intestinal flora. The intestines are filled with digestive microbes and the growth of these can either be retarded or accelerated by the electromagnetic fields that they are in. Retardation will bring about poor digestion and acceleration will bring on excessive gas due to overgrowth inside the intestines. I experienced the gassy overgrowth effect in one of my jobs when I was sitting next to an electrical room daily.

Fertility appears to improve away from wireless technologies. Before trying to get pregnant, I recommend that people clean up their electromagnetic environments to give their children the best chance of going to the full term of 9 months and being born into an environment that is conducive to their healthy development.

Royal Raymond Rife (May 16, 1888 – August 5, 1971) was developing frequencies of energy for medical treatments. He found that certain frequencies would alleviate medical conditions. His work appeared to evolve into what we now know today as transcutaneous electrical nerve stimulation (TENS) devices that are used to heal and radio frequency therapy that produces deep heating in the body tissues and stimulates collagen tightening, repair and regeneration.

The effects of magnetic fields have been noticed in animals. When reviewing the wrf.org article *Magnetic Effects on Living Organisms*, we find:

Regarding sex life and aging the researchers found the following: "...the sex life and the mice and rats we used as controls was considered to be normal. The sex life of the N pole rodents was limited and less active than the controls. It was noted that experiments with the mice, rats and rabbits all resulted in the same percentage of exactness in resulting behavior. The S pole rodents, encompassing all of the above mentioned types, reacted to a far greater sex life with frequent activity. The exposure of the rodents to the S pole energies acted to inspire strength and vigor and when applied to the sex organs encouraged greater development of sperm produced and larger percentages of resultant fertility. This was responsible in part for changing the rodents and animals in their inborn habits, personalities, behavior and reproduction. (Note: Please consult the book for specific details. WRF is merely quoting these sources but not recommending them for human use.) The life span of rodents and animals can be extended up to 50 percent. Mice and rats proved this possibility. In larger animals it has been more difficult to note this due to their normal life span reaching 18 to 25 years, as in the case of cats and dogs."

The hair on the body is likely to be acting like point emitters of ions. Walking around in insulated shoes is likely to have broken much of the energy flow process in the human from the ground into the air. The beneficial health effects of being barefoot on non-electrified soil have been documented in the book "Earthing: The Most Important Health Discovery Ever?".

The womb and placenta may be sources of electrical energy in the body. It has been known for a long time that by subjecting plant soil and roots to electricity can affect their growth. The correct energy stimulates growth and the wrong kind stunts it. The amniotic fluid in the womb is likely to have energies flowing in it that stimulate the growth of the baby and this energy may be generated in the placenta. Placing the womb into abnormal fields of electromagnetic radiation is a really bad idea as it will affect the energy in the womb. Ideally, pregnant women should not be working during their pregnancy due to this effect.

The human body produces significant electromagnetic radiation when moving. Someone passing a stationary human will induce electromagnetic radiation into the resting person. Nikola Tesla documents similar effects when he was developing his research. Indeed, he had noted that an electrical discharge "Flame" that he had generated was affected by his movements, no matter how small they were.

So how does all of this relate to nature?

B. Blake Levitt reports accelerated plant growth and plant defects in her book "Electromagnetic Fields". When reviewing energy levels in the atmosphere and the soil, she states:

What had become known, however, by the end of the eighteenth century was the existence of vast atmospheric electricity and that the soil constantly emits electrically charged particles into the air.

Dr. John Nash Ott had noticed many effects regarding electromagnetic radiation and nature. He had noticed that when a RADAR transmitter had been installed at the local airport that animals that he was filming started to react to it. He timed the rotation period of the RADAR unit and found that it matched a "dance" that the animals were displaying when he filmed them. You can see this in his DVD "Exploring the Spectrum".

Regarding televisions, he had noticed that plants would deform near to them and that animal behaviors were extensively changed when spending long periods of time in front of them. He had also noticed that plants 50 feet away from the televisions would show problems! This matches my research, as I found extensive plant growth defects outdoors in my garden when researching my digital television emissions that cleared up when it was taken out of service.

His research into florescent lights was extensive and he found that plants would deform near to the ends of the florescent light tubes. He also found that animal behaviors changed when they were placed near to the tube ends. His conclusion was that the tube cathodes were emitting X-rays and he developed lead shields that eliminated the growth problems. This is concerning, as most florescent products do not use lead shields on the cathodes.

He found that he could change the sex of offspring of certain animals and fish simply by changing the lighting product that they were exposed to. He could make the offspring 90% male or 90% female simply changing the color temperature of light!

He found that animals that are subjected to unnatural electromagnetic radiation have a tendency to eat their young, even when they have plenty of food. Mankind has significantly altered the electromagnetic environment in the arctic circle through various forms of pollution and polar bears are now being observed to eat their young.

By filtering light with colored filters, it appeared that he could induce impotence into the males! Impotence is on the rise in the human population and may be related to this effect.

He could turn sick animals into healthy animals simply by adding ultraviolet wavelengths of light to the lighting products that they were exposed to. He also noted that sick indoor plants and animals would become healthy simply by moving them outside into natural daylight.

There are no doubts that unnatural radiation exposure damages genetics. Once the genetics have been damaged in many of the world's species we will have entered a new period of evolution that has unknown consequences for humanity. Unfortunately, it is likely that we are in that period today. This is called "Mutating" and Wikipedia states:

In molecular biology and genetics, mutations are changes in a genomic sequence: the DNA sequence of a cell's genome or the DNA or RNA sequence of a virus. They can be defined as sudden and spontaneous changes in the cell. Mutations are caused by radiation, viruses, transposons and mutagenic chemicals, as well as errors that occur during meiosis or DNA replication. They can also be induced by the organism itself, by cellular processes such as hypermutation.

Species that have damaged genetics may actually die out after several generations. It is rather like inbreeding. Once damaged genetics starts to breed, then the damage may start to multiply in each successive generation. It is not unreasonable to think that this fate awaits humanity in the near future. Raising children in unnatural radiation environments is a really bad idea for this reason!

This effect is called:

Extinction Genetics

The interesting thing is, the cellular biologists have already been genetically engineering extinction genetics in seeds. They are developing plants that produce no fertile seeds in order to make farmers completely dependent on purchasing their seed products every year. Extinction genetics is real and it exists today!

The most well preserved human genetics are found in remote areas of heavily forested lands that have populations of humans that have yet to be contacted by the modern human. It is important for the preservation of undamaged human genetics that these areas are turned into international preserves that are kept secure from outside influences. These tribes of people should never be contacted.

Have you ever wondered why the retirement age is set at 65 years of age? It is a number that was developed out of statistics. It was an age where much of the population had died prior to reaching 65 years of age and few were still alive. Something to think about when you are saving for and looking forward to a future retirement! You have a high probability of being extinct before reaching retirement age. Government retirement systems were traditionally low cost programs that few people got to use. That has changed with the radiation exposures that the population have inadvertently received and people are now living longer as a result. Some electromagnetic radiation researchers say that the world government is encouraging the widespread adoption of radio frequency products in order to artificially lower the average life span through induced radiation diseases. While feasible, it is a difficult point to prove.

Today, the modern human is dying from three major factors:

- Heart disease.
- Cancer.
- Brain disease.

This can be seen in the table on the next page.

Top 15 Causes of Death in the U.S. (2007)

Rank	Ages 1–85+	Rank	Ages 1–85+	Rank	Ages 1–85+
1	Heart Disease 615,616	6	Alzheimer's Disease 74,629	11	Septicemia 34,543
2	Malignant Neoplasms 562,795	7	Diabetes Mellitus 71,373	12	Liver Disease 29,158
3	Cerebrovascular 135,814	8	Influenza and Pneumonia 52,492	13	Hypertension 23,963
4	Chronic Lower Respiratory Disease 127,875	9	Nephritis 46,304	14	Parkinson's Disease 20,056
5	Unintentional Injury 122,387	10	Suicide 34,592	15	Homicide 17,984

Data courtesy of CDC

There are no doubts that unnatural electromagnetic radiation exposure can cause all three problems to occur. They are likely to become known as the hallmarks of the man-made electromagnetic death processes as we gain more knowledge in this area. Many reports of heart, brain and cancer conditions are made from people who are subjected to electromagnetic radiation from cell phone towers and Smart/AMR/AMI radiation transmitting utility meters. Indeed, I have personally experienced heart arrhythmia and altered mental functioning induced into me from commonly found electromagnetic fields and that is two out of three! It is reasonable to think that long term exposure to biologically toxic electromagnetic fields that are clearly affecting your health would increase your chances of developing cancer.

Regarding cancer, it is how severe genetic mutations appear in the human. Cancer is a growth of abnormal cells that are replicating into the cancerous growth. Sometimes that replication is controlled by the human immune system and other times it gets out of control and kills the person.

Wikipedia states:

Cancer /ˈkænsər/ (listen), known medically as a malignant neoplasm, is a broad group of various diseases, all involving unregulated cell growth. In cancer, cells divide and grow uncontrollably, forming malignant tumors, and invade nearby parts of the body. The cancer may also spread to more distant parts of the body through the lymphatic system or bloodstream. Not all tumors are cancerous. Benign tumors do not grow uncontrollably, do

324

not invade neighboring tissues, and do not spread throughout the body.

Skin cancer is one of the more prevalent forms of cancer. Man-made electromagnetic radiation exposures should be expected to increase these levels, as the skin is the primary defense for the human to this unnatural biological toxin.

Depression is increasing in the world population and it appears to be coming from exposure to radiation sources. Lighting products appear to create it, as does dirty electricity. Certain types of electronic products are toxic and exposure to these may induce it.

Depression is likely caused by cellular problems in the human mind and body when exposed to toxic sources of electromagnetic radiation.

It is well known that life expectancy is modified according to radiation exposure. The next graph shows what I have been able to ascertain about how this occurs.

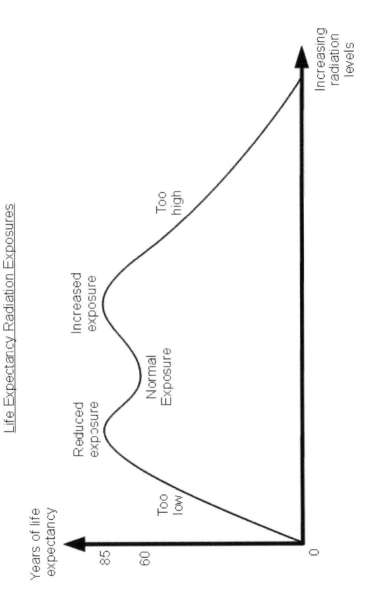

I call the effect of changing the electromagnetic environment into a form that cannot sustain life:

Extinction Energy

Today, we are witnessing the greatest threat to the survival of mankind emerging, and that is:

Species Extinction

We have entered the next extinction period in recorded history and it is man-made. Wikipedia states:

The Anthropocene is a recent and informal geologic chronological term that serves to mark the evidence and extent of human activities that have had a significant global impact on the Earth's ecosystems. The term was coined by ecologist Eugene F. Stoermer but has been widely popularized by the Nobel Prize-winning atmospheric chemist Paul Crutzen, who regards the influence of human behavior on the Earth's atmosphere in recent centuries as so significant as to constitute a new geological era for its lithosphere.

In 2008 a proposal was presented to the Stratigraphy Commission of the Geological Society of London to make the Anthropocene a formal unit of geological time. A large majority of that Stratigraphy Commission decided the proposal had merit and should therefore be examined further. Steps are being taken by independent working groups of scientists from various geological societies to determine if the Anthropocene will be formally accepted into the Geological Time Scale.

Wow! We have the privilege of having being born into a massive extinction period of the Earth's history. Unfortunately for the human, it is at the very top of the food chain and if the food chain starts to collapse, then it will be greatly affected. The food chain for the human has started that process and it has been noticed in recent years that the extinction process for the honey bee is well underway. It is called "Bee Colony Collapse" and it started several years ago. It is widely acknowledged that human extinction would be tied to that of the honey bee.

Wikipedia states:

Colony collapse disorder (CCD) is a phenomenon in which worker bees from a beehive or European honey bee colony abruptly disappear. While such disappearances have occurred throughout the history of apiculture, the term colony collapse disorder was first applied to a drastic rise in the number of disappearances of Western honey bee colonies in North America in late 2006. Colony collapse is significant because many agricultural crops worldwide are pollinated by bees.

European beekeepers observed similar phenomena in Belgium, France, the Netherlands, Greece, Italy, Portugal, and Spain, and initial reports have also come in from Switzerland and Germany, albeit to a lesser degree while the Northern Ireland Assembly received reports of a decline greater than 50%. Possible cases of CCD have also been reported in Taiwan since April 2007.

The quote on the next page sums up the situation that humanity now finds itself in.

"If the bee disappears from the surface of the earth, man would have no more than four years to live." - Unknown

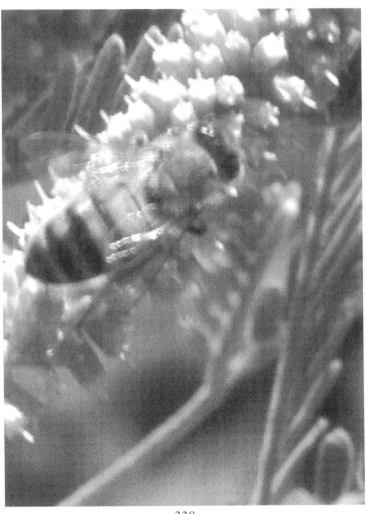

The effects of global warming and climate change will be catastrophic to the Earth and humanity. There are no doubts that it is caused by the emissions from the era that is currently documented as the "Industrial Revolution". Amongst the biggest fossil fuel polluters in the world are the electrical utilities.

The electrical utilities are getting increasingly desperate to source their fossil fuels and we are seeing the more difficult resources being developed. The controversial "fracking" technique is now being used throughout the USA to tap into the shale to generate gas. There is blatantly willful negligent behavior taking place in this industry where peoples contaminated drinking well water is being denied. Despite the public exposure of this in the films "Gasland" and "Gasland Part 2", the industry is still claiming that the fracking technique is safe. One has to wonder how this can possibly occur when innocent people are able to set their drinking water on fire due to so much gas contamination from the fracking technique!

One of the desperate measures being undertaken is the adoption of solar and wind power by the utilities. Both of these technologies have issues that are currently emerging. In the wind power industry, the following documentation has arrived in recent years:

- The Wind Farm Scam by John Etherington.
- Wind Turbine Syndrome: A Report on a Natural Experiment by Nina Pierpont.
- Windfall (2010): A film by Laura Israel.

Between them, they do a good job of explaining the factual problems in both energy production and the detrimental human health and nature issues around the wind turbines.

Solar photovoltaics has issues as well, and these are currently emerging:

- Engineers and designers who do not understand solar photovoltaics nor the optical environment that they are designing systems for.

- Construction permits being issued by officials who do not understand solar photovoltaics nor optics.

- Poorly designed systems may overload and go on fire.

- DC arcing and DC fires as equipment ages and breaks down.

- Inverter electromagnetic field emissions.

- System electromagnetic field emissions into the human environment.

- Unnatural solar radiation levels in the human environment from solar reflections. A solar power worker may develop a strange form of radiation sickness from working outdoors around these systems.

- Solar glare.

- Increased thermal activity above the system.

- Harmonics.

- Dirty electricity.

- Intermittent power production.

- Daytime only power production.

- Seasonal power production.

- Installation into environments that are unsuited to the technology.

- Stray voltage/current/frequency exposures.

- The industry staying relatively silent about the problems.

I can tell you that during working full time at a very large utility solar photovoltaic power plant for a couple of months, my health went terrible. My body was filled with aches and pains, and my sleep cycle was off. My concentration was off and my ability to handle stressful situations was compromised. My senses would not be working right and I found that I would make simple mistakes for no rational reason. I occasionally would find myself in a state of confusion when trying to do simple tasks. My mating cycle was being triggered. The solar power plant was producing high levels of electronically generated harmonic energy and this was definitely a factor in the health issues that I was seeing.

After I left the electronic utility power plant, I noticed that my memory was having issues as well. I could not remember telephone numbers, alarm codes, computer passwords, and my ability to do basic mathematics was compromised. It slowly improved after performing the radiation detoxification process. It took about a year for things to significantly improve from the toxic exposures of the system.

This appeared to be a form of dementia and this leads me to conclude that dementia may actually be curable.

I had noticed aggression, fatigue, confusion and memory problems in the staff at the site. In conversations with them, they were also reporting insomnia, general aches and pains.

The solar reflection problem is shown in the next picture and this raises the solar radiation levels in the human environment to unnaturally high levels.

The reflections from solar modules raise the radiation levels significantly in the human environment.

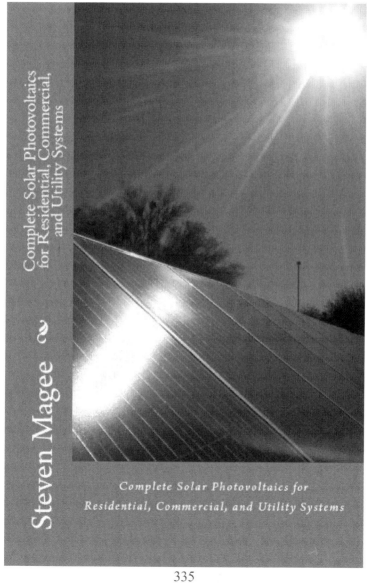

Some of these problems also apply to wind energy systems. In particular, electronic power generation by inverters is a feature shared by both. Electronic power generation into the grid is relatively new and the long term human health consequences of electronically generated harmonic energy are not yet fully understood.

While alternate energy systems appear appealing, they quite often are installed for public relations and investor purposes, rather than to generate significant quantities of energy into the utility grid.

The current generation of solar and wind power systems generally introduce instability into the electrical utility grid system with their intermittent power generation characteristics and electronically generated harmonic energy. Generally, there has to be a peaking gas turbine plant near to the very large utility installations to offset these unstable energy generation systems. Unfortunately, these peaking power plants are the lowest efficiency way of generating fossil fuel energy into the utility grid. A wind or solar farm combined with a peaking power plant may not actually save any fossil fuel emissions when compared to a high efficiency conventional power plant. In some cases, they may actually use more energy!

This is evidenced by the global energy consumption increasing annually. The time has come to face reality and that a continuation of the current insanity of polluting the atmosphere must come to end. The reality is that we must significantly reduce pollution and the only effective way we know how to do this today is to stop consuming energy.

It is interesting to note that there was no electrical energy industry just over a century ago and everything worked well. Energy consumption is comparable to drug addiction. You do not need the drugs, but you take them anyway. You know that they will eventually kill you, but you are addicted and unable to change your ways.

The addition of the fossil fuel emissions to the atmosphere appears to have changed the sunsets from white to the yellows, oranges, and reds that we have today. This can be observed when reviewing works of art of Sun and Moon sets from several hundred years ago. This means that the fossil fuel emissions have changed the atmospheric solar radiation transmission and, by association, the electromagnetic radiation environment. Air pollution affects many forms of electromagnetic radiation and how they are transmitted through the atmosphere.

You should be concerned when the Sun does not appear white. This can also occur when the Sun is viewed through city pollution and emissions from chimneys.

The next page shows the fossil fuel sunset from Kitt Peak Observatory in Sells, Arizona. This orange sunset was taken at an altitude of approximately 6,875 feet. It probably would have been a white sunset several hundred years ago.

The atmospheric filtered orange sunset from Kitt Peak.

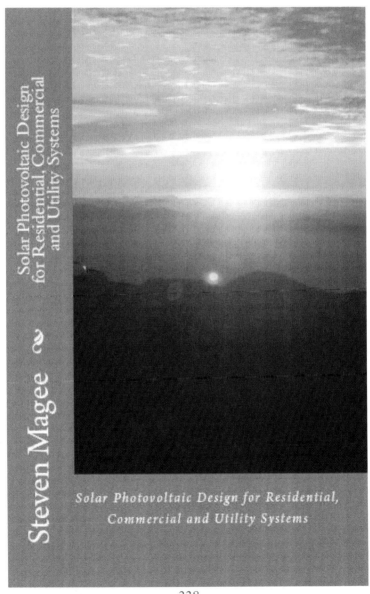

Massachusetts Institute of Technology (MIT) says:

"Most of the computer scenarios found population and economic growth continuing at a steady rate until about 2030. But without "drastic measures for environmental protection," the scenarios predict the likelihood of a population and economic crash..."There is a very clear warning bell being rung here," Turner said. "We are not on a sustainable trajectory."

Did you know that fossil fuel pollution may bring about the extinction wavelength of light and extinction energy? Did you know climate change and global warming change the electromagnetic radiation environment? It is probably only a matter of time before environmental conditions move outside of the long term human survival range as global atmospheric pollution continues to accelerate.

Time is rapidly running out on humanity!

"The greatest discoveries of science have always been those that forced us to rethink our beliefs about the universe and our place in it."
Robert L. Park

Health Statistics

Dr Samuel Milham reports in his book "Dirty Electricity" that over 50 residential and over 100 occupational studies now associate power frequency magnetic field exposures with cancer. As such, you should be aware of your electrical environment.

He states that the following professions have increased mortality due to leukemia, lymphoma, and brain tumors:

- **Power station workers.**
- **Electricians.**
- **Power line workers.**
- **Telephone line workers.**
- **Aluminum workers.**
- **Radio and TV repair workers.**
- **Welders.**

He found that amateur radio operators have an increase in mortality due to lymphoma and acute myloid leukemia which relates to the power level that they are licensed for.

He sums up his findings in his book "Dirty Electricity" with:

__The price we have paid for the convenience of electricity in morbidity and mortality since the early 1900's almost defies quantification.__

The Berenson-Allen Center for Noninvasive Brain Stimulation knows how electromagnetic fields can affect the brain. They are using the following techniques that Wikipedia states:

- *Transcranial direct current stimulation (tDCS) is a form of neurostimulation which uses constant, low current delivered directly to the brain area of interest via small electrodes:*

- *Transcranial magnetic stimulation (TMS) is a noninvasive method to cause depolarization or hyperpolarization in the neurons of the brain. TMS uses electromagnetic induction to induce weak electric currents using a rapidly changing magnetic field; this can cause activity in specific or general parts of the brain with minimal discomfort, allowing for study of the brain's functioning and interconnections. A variant of TMS, repetitive transcranial magnetic stimulation (rTMS) has been tested as a treatment tool for various neurological and psychiatric disorders including migraines, strokes, Parkinson's disease, dystonia, tinnitus and depression.*

When reviewing their website *http://tmslab.org/index.php*, we find:

We are a world leader in research and development, clinical application, and teaching of noninvasive brain stimulation. We use noninvasive brain stimulation to gain novel insights into the human brain and mind.

Our work has been fundamental in establishing noninvasive brain stimulation as a valuable tool in clinical and fundamental neuroscience, improving the technology and its integration with several brain-imaging methodologies, and helping to create the field of therapeutic noninvasive brain stimulation. We are committed to provide education and training on the use of noninvasive brain stimulation for both clinical practice and research.

Our clinical program offers noninvasive brain stimulation for diagnostic applications and treatment of a variety of neuropsychiatric disorders such as depression, schizophrenia, epilepsy, dystonia, Parkinson's disease, chronic pain, epilepsy, autism, and the neurorehabilitation of motor function, cognition, and language after stroke or traumatic brain injury.

When you look at the USA you find some interesting observations that have been noted by researchers.

Obesity is on the rise. When reviewing the Yahoo News article *Mom's obesity tied to kids' autism, development* we find:

Meanwhile, Krakowiak and her colleagues note that nearly 60 percent of U.S. women of childbearing age (20-39 years) are overweight, one-third are obese and 16 percent have so-called metabolic syndrome -- a constellation of symptoms, including high blood pressure and insulin resistance, that raise heart disease risk.

When reviewing the Arizona Daily Star article *CDC: 1 in 64 kids in AZ has autism* we find:

Nationally, autism spectrum disorders are almost five times more common among boys than girls, the study found.

The rate for boys in Arizona is 1 in 40, and the rate for girls is 1 in 185.

Autism is a brain disorder that affects a person's ability to communicate, to reason and to interact with others. It affects individuals differently and to varying degrees of severity, and it is often found in combination with other disabilities.

The terms "autism" and "autism spectrum disorder" are often used interchangeably. Among conditions included on the autism spectrum are Asperger's, pervasive developmental disorder and Rett syndrome.

The number of children identified with autism spectrum disorder ranged from 1 in 210 children in Alabama to 1 in 47 children in Utah.

The largest increases were among Hispanic and black children.

343

When reviewing *breastcancer.org* we find:

About 1 in 8 U.S. women (just under 12%) will develop invasive breast cancer over the course of her lifetime.

For women in the U.S., breast cancer death rates are higher than those for any other cancer, besides lung cancer.

The rural Chinese people have noticed that breast cancer is almost none existent in the countryside and is prevalent in the cities. They call it *The Rich Woman's Disease.*

Insomnia is prevalent in the population and this generally leads to these people taking sleep medications. In one study of people who were taking sleep medications it was found that they were 5 times more likely to die than those who did not. Heavy users of sleep medications were more likely to develop cancer. Insomnia has definite links to certain types electrical lighting products and electromagnetic radiation exposures.

The photosynthesis effects play an important role in the human body, especially in childhood development. Vitamin D deficiency is known to cause bone growth defects and affects calcium absorption. It also increases the likelihood of bone fractures. Vitamin B12 now appears to be linked to vitamin D deficiency and it affects the brain and spinal cord. It appears that Autism is linked to unnatural light exposures as B12 vitamin injections are now being used with success to treat Autism. When reviewing the livestrong.com article *Methyl B12 Shots And Autism*, we find:

Neubrander reports that treatment with methyl B12 injections leads to increased executive functions, such as cognition and awareness, better language skills, greater emotional responsiveness, and improved socialization and play skills. Neubrander indicates that around 90 percent of his own patients have demonstrated improved symptoms with this treatment.

Regarding crime, the USA has 760 prisoners per 100,000 people in the population. This equates to 0.76% of the USA citizens are in jail! It is the highest jail rate in the modern world. The USA has 5% of the world's population and 25% of the world's prisoners.

Social degradation has been noticed by many researchers and it appears to be getting worse with time. The modern human is losing the social skills of honesty, integrity, compassion, empathy, caring for the future of the next generation, and the ability to read and understand the social situations that it finds itself in.

When reviewing the BBC News report *Many adults think children are 'feral'*, we find:

Of the more than 2,000 people questioned by ICM Research, 44% said young people were becoming feral.

Barnado's chief executive Anne Marie Carrie said it was "depressing" so many were ready to give up on children.

The survey revealed that:

- *49% agreed children are beginning to behave like animals.*

- *Almost 47% thought youngsters were angry, violent and abusive.*

- *One in four said those who behaved badly were beyond help by the age of 10.*

- *Whilst 36% thought children who get into trouble need help, 38% disagreed.*

When you examine the death statistics in the USA, you find that the death rate takes off after the age of thirty. Cancer and heart related problems are what the majority of middle aged people die of. I am sure that you would agree with me that people should not be dying in their thirties or forties. People who are dying so young have likely been exposed to excessive environmental toxins. This is shown on the next page.

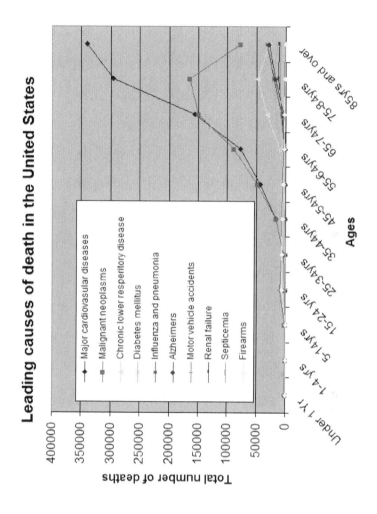

One has to wonder if these are all problems caused by various kinds of electromagnetic radiation exposures?

The interesting thing about electromagnetic radiation is that the people who understand it the least are the medical profession! Indeed, a hospital is regarded by many as one of the most toxic environments that you can go into.

Their scanners generally use various forms of electromagnetic radiation to peer inside the body. The building will be lit by electronic florescent lighting products. The medical devices may be emitting large amounts of EMI. There may be a television right next to your bed or on the other side of the wall to your bed. The window is probably low-E coated double glazed glass. The security doors may be using radio frequency identification devices (RFID). The building wiring probably has dirty electricity on it. The communications devices in the building may be wireless transmitters. On the roof there may be many high powered communication transmitters. Indeed, I have noticed multiple cell phone towers right next door to a hospital in Tucson! It is an interesting concept to have radiation transmitting devices next to a hospital that are known to significantly increase the illness rates in people who live within a quarter of a mile of them.

The roof of a hospital is shown in the next picture. Note the extensive range of communication antennas. You would not want to be spending extended time in the top floors of this building.

It is normal to see many radiation transmitting systems on the roof of most modern hospitals.

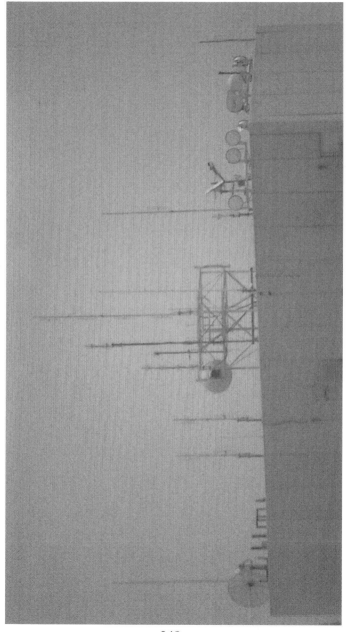

The big thing that you will notice about a hospital is the smell! Excessive use of cleaning products is harmful to the human mind and body and will out-gas many toxins into the air. As such, the air is extremely contaminated inside a hospital. I noticed that I always had lung pains when I worked for thirteen years in a hospital and they cleared up when I left for my next position!

The USA medical system is ran for maximum profits at the expense of the sick people. The medical system has a long history of bankrupting many sick Americans who have had to use it. When reviewing the aarp.org article *5 Myths About Canada's Health Care System*, we find:

...Third of the Americans surveyed reported that...they didn't go to the doctor when sick...about one in five of the Americans surveyed had struggled to pay or were unable to pay their medical bills in the preceding year...We're spending way more on health care than any other country, and for all that money we're getting at best middling results.

When you realize that the medical profession has chosen not to understand the very basics of the human genetic environment, it does make you understand how these problems have occurred. These are all very simple problems that have very simple fixes. They are all caused by:

Incorrect Environmental Conditions

And the preventative measure for these health problems is:

Correct Environmental Conditions

When reviewing the npr.org article *Why Getting Grimy As A Child Can Make For A Healthier Life*, we find:

We've known for a while that people who grow up on farms are less likely to have ailments related to the immune system than people who grow up in cities. Those include asthma, allergies, inflammatory bowel disease and multiple sclerosis.

The human has the genetics of an outdoor forest animal. By realizing this and increasing your outdoor exposures in a green environment with a tree canopy and reducing your exposures to electromagnetic radiation sources will clear up the majority of health issues. Eating natural organic food and drinking mineral water is essential to human health. Being fit and muscular is the natural physical state of the human. The human is also supposed to have an annual detoxification cycle in wintertime and the restoration of this cycle may return you to good health. Simple!

"It is horrifying that we have to fight our own government to save the environment."

Ansel Adams

Avoiding EMR

If we take a look at the history of electromagnetic radiation we can see that there are definite steps in the progress of it throughout society:

- 1800's-1860's: Telegraph development marks the start of widespread man-made electromagnetic interference exposure in the general population.

- 1870's: Edison develops the phonograph and starts manufacturing light bulbs.

- 1880's: Edison and Tesla are developing their electrical distribution systems. Edison sets up the first electrical utility using a 110 volt direct current (DC) system in New York City.

- 1890's: Oil and gas were starting to replace coal and wood. X-rays discovered. Tesla sets up the first alternating current (AC) utility in Niagara Falls.

- 1900's: Cars and airplanes were developing with batteries and electrical ignition systems.

- 1910's: Radio is being developed. First World War. Nikola Tesla's mental health is degrading and he is having financial problems.

- 1920's: Widespread adoption of Tesla's alternating current electrical system in cities. Leukemia is appearing in the population. The mass population is being exposed to electric lights and cinema.

- 1930's: Widespread adoption of radio. RADAR and jet engine is in development. Male impotence is

being documented in RADAR workers. Thomas
Edison dies.

- 1940's: Widespread adoption of the alternating
  current (AC) electrical system in farming
  communities. Second World War. Development of
  nuclear bombs and worldwide dispersal of man-
  made fall-out radiation. Nikola Tesla dies.

- 1950's: Development of the transistor and nuclear
  power. Extensive air testing of nuclear bombs and
  worldwide radiation fallout. Dr. John Nash Ott is
  discovering many detrimental health effects of
  electromagnetic radiation.

- 1960's: Widespread adoption of televisions and
  cars. The modern computer is being developed.
  The Space industry is being developed. The
  medical profession is trying to understand organ
  failure. Nuclear bomb testing moved underground
  to prevent worldwide radiation dispersal. Dr. John
  Nash Ott is discovering X-ray emissions from
  florescent lights and televisions.

- 1970's: Widespread use of digital watches and
  calculators. Adoption of international jet travel.
  Many communications satellites are now in orbit.
  Smooth float glass is becoming common in
  buildings. Color television became popular. Dr.
  John Nash Ott is discovering that electrical lighting
  products are changing the gender of animals and
  plants.

- 1980's: Widespread adoption of home and business
  computers, video games, video recorders and
  portable cassette players. Typical microprocessor
  speed of 1Mhz. Satellite television is in homes, as
  are radioactive ionizing smoke detectors. Diabetes
  is widespread. Cell phone towers are being

constructed. Dr. John Nash Ott is discovering that the new electronic products are causing health problems in humans. Florescent lighting products are inducing cancer into his laboratory rats.

- 1990's: Widespread adoption of digital electronics into the home and workplace. Typical processor speed of 10Mhz. Cordless home and business phones that use radio frequencies are becoming popular. Coated double glazed glass is becoming commonplace in homes and businesses. RADAR systems are in use in commercial applications and weather forecasting. Autism is starting to become prevalent. Construction of International Space Station (ISS) is started. Rapid construction of cell phone towers is significantly raising the radiation levels. Dr. John Nash Ott is failing in his efforts to get his findings out to the mainstream population, media organizations will not report it.

- 2000's: Internet was widely adopted and much of commerce became conducted using it. Laptop computers and cellphones became popular. Typical processor speed of 100Mhz. Ionizing smoke detectors are installed in every bedroom. Electrical outlets are now installed every ten feet in homes. Obesity epidemic underway. Bee colonies are collapsing around the world. Fraudulent invasions of countries. Dr. John Nash Ott dies after much of his work is willfully ignored by the government, corporations, media, and research institutions.

- 2010's: GPS systems, tablet computers and smart phones became popular. Almost all young children now have cellphones, computers, and electrical and electronic toys. Typical processor speed of 1 Ghz. Breast cancer is affecting 1 in 8 women. Almost all

types of cancer are increasing. Autism and
Attention Deficit Disorder (ADD) are widespread.
Atmospheric carbon dioxide is double the historical
records. Construction of the International Space
Station is completed and it is the largest man-made
object in orbit. The Earth is ringed in thousands of
man-made satellites that are regularly eclipsing the
Sun. The sky is filled with chemical trails from jet
aircraft that linger for hours. Cirrus clouds have
become prevalent. Cell phone coverage of 99% of
the USA population is achieved with many people
in multiple cell phone system transmission areas.
Homes and workplaces have been turned into high
powered antenna parks with the installation of
radiation transmitting Smart/AMR/AMI utility
meters and people are getting sick from them. The
next generation of weather RADAR systems is
installed into USA cities. The human
electromagnetic radiation environment has never
existed in the history of the world. The USA is
calling itself "The Greatest Nation on Earth".

As we can see, electromagnetic interference has been
constantly changing over the last two centuries to the point
where we are immersed in electromagnetic interference
fields that are a soup of various forms of radiation. The
biggest man-made experiment on the Earth is in full swing
and you are a part of it!

As Dr. John Nash Ott reports in his books on the subject,
the media would not report his findings to the general
public. Nor would the corporations that he interacted with.
This makes complete sense when you realize that the two
are linked. The flow of media content to the mass

population is controlled by just a few corporate entities. When reviewing the nationofchange.org article *Illusion of Choice*, we find:

Media has never been more consolidated. 6 media giants now control a staggering 90% of what we read, watch or listen to.

During the course of developing this book, I ran many experiments on my own mind and body to see how it reacted around electrical, electronic and wireless systems. I can tell you that withdrawal symptoms can occur from removing the following exposures to the human mind and body:

- Utility Power lines.
- Dirty electricity.
- Inverter systems.
- Dirty electrical and electronic products.
- Sitting too close to a television (in all directions).
- Computer systems.
- Certain artificial lighting products.
- High powered transmitters.
- Cell phones.
- Grounding systems.

When evaluating your environment for toxic exposures, you should start at your bedroom and work your way out to the street. Look at your workplace next. Your daily commute may be exposing you to toxins and pay attention to power lines, cell phone towers, and transmitters along your route. After this you should look into transmitting devices near to both your home and workplace. http://www.antennasearch.com/ will allow you to get a good idea of how many transmitters are in the area. A search on the White House reveals almost 600 antenna systems nearby!

The biggest source of toxins to your mind and body are usually found in the areas that you spend the most amount of time. Your home is the top place for that exposure!

The more electrical, electronic and wireless products that you have in your environment, the more likely it is that you may become ill.

Simplicity is healthy!

It is important to be aware of the locations of electrical, electronic and wireless equipment in both your home and work environments. Some things to pay attention to are:

- Know the locations of electrical fuse boards and utility meters and stay away from them.

- Avoid spending time near computer server rooms, electrical rooms, mechanical rooms and elevator shafts.

- Know where the wireless transmitting devices are and stay away from them.

- Stay away from electrical transformers. You should be aware of their locations and avoid being on the floor directly above or below them.

- Stay away from electrical generator rooms.

- If utility power lines and poles are near to the building, stay out of that area.

- On your commute to work, pay attention to the locations and type of power lines along your route. Choose routes that avoid having power lines running along them. Drive in the lane furthest away from them.

- If there is a streetlight that shines light into your bedroom, make sure that you have a blackout blind on the window that blocks out all of the light from it.

So what is the cure for electromagnetic hypersensitivity? The only known cure is to return your environment back to a natural levels of electromagnetic radiation.

The main thing that you can do is reduce your exposure by switching off as much of your electrical, electronic and wireless products as possible. You should also identify how much electromagnetic interference each of your products emits. A simple AM radio tuned to static (no radio station) can detect most electromagnetic interference fields and they are strongest at the equipment and fade with distance.

Clear your home from these products and just have the products that you really need. Naturally, your bedrooms should be free of any electromagnetic interference producing equipment. If you are going to use electromagnetic interference producing equipment, then you should be using low electromagnetic interference versions of it wherever possible. You should consider switching off the electrical circuit breakers for rooms that you do not use and also the bedrooms. It is a good idea not to be exposed to AC electrical fields while you are sleeping.

On radial electrical circuits for outlets, you can install a switch at the first electrical socket that enables you to turn the circuit on and off as you need it. You can also split the circuit with a switch and have some sockets on permanently, and others switched on as they are needed. Once you have installed switches onto your circuits, you should get into the habit of turning off circuits that you are not using. This is shown in the next photgraph.

Clean up your bedroom. You should not have electricity in your bedroom nor electrical, electronic nor wireless products. You should avoid sleeping on a metal mattress and have a foam one instead, preferably a natural latex one. Most cellular damage occurs during sleep due to the cellular regeneration processes taking place during this time.

After I switched off the majority of AC circuits in my home, I noticed the following withdrawal symptoms occurring:

- Aching joints and bones.

- Fatigue.

- Headaches.

- Difficulty in waking up in the morning.

The symptoms cleared up after approximately one week.

Installing a switch at the first radial socket enables you to turn the circuit on or off as you require it. When it is off, it will reduce the electromagnetic fields within your home.

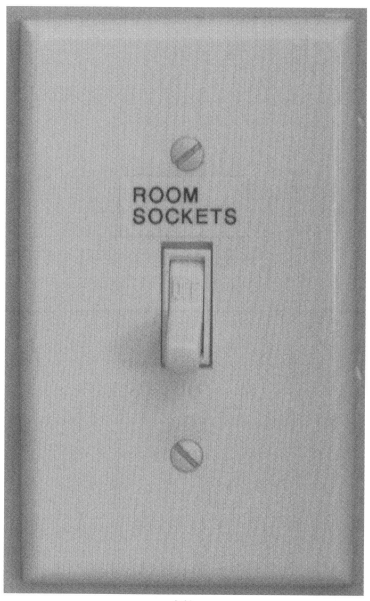

Have an electrician check your electrical ground, plumbing ground, conductive flooring, water systems, drains and garden for stray voltage/current/frequency and dirty electricity effects.

If you are serious about eliminating the sources of electromagnetic interference then you may want to obtain the following items of test equipment to aid with diagnosing problems (My test equipment is in the brackets):

- A portable, battery powered analogue AM radio (Sharper Image Model GFSI-0100).

- A digital multimeter with a minimum and maximum feature (Amprobe 5XP-A).

- A magnetic field, electric field, and microwave field meter (TriField Model 100XE).

- A battery powered oscilloscope with a Fast Fourier Transform function (FFT) (Owon PDS 5022S).

- A three axis radio frequency meter 10 MHz to 8 GHz (Tenmars TM-196).

- A battery powered RADAR detector (Whistler XTR 445).

- A camcorder with high speed video (slow motion) and time lapse functions (JVC Everio GZ-EX210).

You should make yourself aware of the peak load times of the electrical systems in your area and see if they coincide with health problems occurring:

- Air conditioning loads of summertime.

- Heating loads of wintertime.

- Industrial area load peaks are 08:00 to 17:00.

- Residential area load peaks are 16:00 to 20:00.

- Solar power system peaks are two hours after sunrise through to two hours before sunset on a clear and sunny day. On a day with broken clouds, they will produce rapid energy swings on the electricity system. You may get the poorest quality electricity on cloudy days.

- Wind power peaks will coincide with the rising wind speed in the area. Wind power systems generally do not make much power below 20 MPH wind speeds. They should generate significant electrical power above 30 MPH. You may get the poorest quality electricity at the lowest wind speeds.

You should also pay attention to where you spend time and how you feel in those environments. A long drive may bring on symptoms from exposure to car electromagnetic interference and pollution. Time spent at your job may bring on symptoms from either Sick Building Syndrome or pollution that your job exposes you to. Your employer may be avoiding informing you of known hazards of your job, as they may have seen the same thing with previous employees and know that the job is hazardous to human health. You may be the latest employee getting sick out of the many people who came before you!

The design of your home may be affecting your health. Small homes with little rooms bring you closer to the electrical cables. Low ceilings do the same. All of the electrical, electronic and wireless products will be closer to you as well.

It is a well known fact that poorer people are sicker than richer people and the size of the homes is probably a factor.

You should avoid using electric blankets, as they will put a very large AC voltage onto your mind and body. Even when they are off, they may induce voltage into you from the neutral and grounding system cables. The neutral and grounding cables may emit a wide range of frequencies into the human.

Electromagnetic interference is proven to affect cellular development and it is especially important to identify exposures in babies and developing children. Cellular development probably has far more to do with electromagnetic radiation exposure than any other factor. You should characterize the radio frequency environment of your home and sleep in the low radiation rooms. The lowest radiation rooms are the ones where your children should be sleeping, as they are the most vulnerable to the biologically harmful effects.

It is an unfortunate state of affairs that we find ourselves having to do the governments job of protecting ourselves from known harm. Electrical, electronic and wireless equipment should never have been allowed into the home or workplace that may cause harm to human health. It is a clear sign that self regulation by industries does not work and that profits have been put before human health. With the recent environmental disasters of Hurricane Katrina in

2005, the BP Deepwater Horizon oil spill in 2010 and the Fukushima nuclear power plant disaster of 2011 we can see that the government systems of public protection are failing.

In this "modern" society, it is clear that you are responsible for your own health. Ultimately, if you have EHS, you may have to move to the countryside to a known low electromagnetic radiation area if you are unable to clean up your environment sufficiently. Trees are excellent at suppressing electromagnetic interference due to their effective grounding. They essentially are nature's version of the Faraday cage that is used to suppress electromagnetic interference in the engineering field.

An interesting fact that bears some thought are the differences that were observed in Edison and Tesla. Edison was developing a direct current (DC) electrical system and Tesla was developing an alternating current (AC) system. Edison was regarded as a respected businessman, while Tesla was regarded as a mad scientist. It is quite possible that the mental issues that Tesla displayed had come from exposure to his work with alternating current. Direct current that Edison was working with does not transmit through the air as well. Both men lived into their 80's and Edison was experimenting with dietary intake towards the end of his life, presumably to cure his ailments. Perhaps Edison had become a victim of exposure to Tesla's alternating current system, the very system that he had lobbied against as being a danger to human health!

It is unfortunate that these electromagnetic interference effects have occurred and we may now have widespread electrical poisoning in the modern world. An

electrically poisoned human is not going to think normally nor function normally. When you observe the modern population you can see that there are many different personalities around, many of which do not appear to be normal and it is probably a sign of poisoning.

Humans are displaying an addiction to electrical energy that appears to be like drug addiction. It rules their lives. Humans should be weaned off electrical energy consumption in order to reduce this unnatural dependance that has been formed. Homes should have trees placed around them to help keep them cool and reduce the air conditioning loads on the electrical grid. Ideally, homes should be located under the tree canopy.

To sum up, here are the suspected human health hazards of electricity:

- Direct contact with electricity system live conductors can cause electric shock, electrical burns and possibly death.

- Corroded utility neutrals may shock and cause electrocution.

- A surge in stray voltage may cause human electrocution in swimming pools and wet areas.

- Long term exposure to AC stray voltage/current/frequency may cause human health to degrade.

- Long term exposure to electric fields may cause human health to degrade.

- Long term exposure to magnetic fields above 2 mill-gauss may cause human health to degrade.

- Long term exposure to radio or microwave fields may cause human health to degrade.

- Long term exposure to an ion field imbalance may cause human health to degrade.

- Long term exposure to power lines may cause human health to degrade.

- Long term exposure to electrostatic fields may cause human health to degrade.

- Long term exposure to electricity that contains harmonics and various frequencies (dirty electricity) may cause human health to degrade.

- Nighttime exposure may be a higher risk, due to radio waves transmitting better during this time.

- Long term exposure to electrical lighting may cause human health to degrade.

Products that are documented by electromagnetic radiation researchers for toxic effects on the human include:

- WiFi.

- Wireless products.

- Cell Phones.

- Products with electrically grounded metal cases.

- Anti-static devices.

- Microwave ovens.

- Electric appliances.

- Laptop computers.

- Televisions.

- Computer monitors.

- Florescent lights.

- Compact florescent lights (CFL).

- Light emitting diode lights (LED).

- Gas discharge lights of all types.

- Power poles and lines.

- Cell phone towers.

- Transmitters.

More details on this subject can be found in the following books:

The health effects of the AC electricity system can be found in "Dirty Electricity: Electrification and the Diseases of Civilization." by Samuel Milham MD MPH. He notes that Leukemia is almost unknown in Africa where there is minimal electrification and the disease appears to be following the progress of electrification. It was unknown by the world medical profession until the 1920's when electricity started to become commonplace.

"Electrocution of America: Is Your Utility Company Out to Kill You?" by Russ Allen documents the problems of stray voltage/current/frequency.

The Earth's ground is now very different and more on this subject can be found in the book "Earthing: The Most

Important Health Discovery Ever?" by Clinton Ober, Stephen T. Sinatra MD and Martin Zucker.

Documentation regarding the rise of electromagnetic interference pollution can be found in the following books

- "Cross Currents: The Perils of Electropollution" by Dr. Robert O. Becker.
- "Electromagnetic Fields: A Consumer's Guide to the Issue and How to Protect Ourselves" by B. Blake Levitt.
- "The Invisible Disease: The Dangers of Environmental Illnesses Caused by Electromagnetic Fields and Chemical Emissions" by Gunni Nordstrom.
- "The Force: Living Safely in a World of Electromagnetic Pollution." by Lyn McClean.
- "Silent Fields" and "Dirty Electricity and Electromagnetic Radiation" by Donna Fisher.

Biological defects associated with electromagnetic radiation can be found in "Light, Radiation, and You." by John N. Ott.

Human health issues in the electronics industry is well documented in "Challenging the Chip: Labor Rights and Environmental Justice in the Global Electronics Industry." by Ted Smith, David A. Sonnenfeld, David Naguib Pellow, and Jim Hightower.

Dr. Magda Havas has an excellent electromagnetic interference (EMI) website at:

www.magdahavas.com

Stray voltage reducing products are available and a popular product is the "Ronk Blocker" from Ronk Electrical Industries.

http://www.ronkelectrical.com/Blocker%201-21.pdf

For detecting dirty electricity, Stetzer Electric have developed the "STETZERiZER Meter".

https://www.stetzerelectric.com/store/stetzerizer-microsurge-meter/

A nice list of research papers about "Dirty Electricity" and the effects on human health can be found at:

http://www.stetzerelectric.com/researchPaper/list.

"All the things that human beings suffer from are how their environment treats them, and how the elements of their planet affects their mind and body - like radiation, cancer, and all."

Ornette Coleman.

Better Construction

The incorrect construction of homes is a large part of the health problems in society. As soon as you see the words "Energy Star" or "Green" you should be concerned! There has been little thought put into home and office construction that is based on correct human environmental conditions. The human has the genetics of an outdoor forest animal and the further you change your home and office from that of a forest environment, the more likely it is that you will get sick.

The forest has the following attributes:

- A tree canopy.
- Nature modification of light.
- Lots of plants.
- Clean flowing, naturally mineralized water.
- Organic food.
- No pollution.
- Recycles everything.
- Naturally regulates the solar radiation environment.
- Naturally regulates the humidity.
- Naturally regulates the temperature.
- Very low levels of electromagnetic radiation.
- Naturally supports the life within it.

- Ionizes the air.

For the humans to mimic nature, what should they do? Keep your environment as close to natural levels as possible. Here are some ideas:

- Construct the home in a natural area free of man-made electromagnetic radiation.

- Build the home in the center of the land.

- Build the home under the tree canopy.

- Keep to single story construction.

- Use natural materials to construct the home.

- Use underground utilities.

- Mount the fuse board and electrical meter to the furthest point from the home on the garage wall.

- Design the home around the electrical products that will be in the home. Do not put chairs or beds near to the electrical products or on the other side of the walls from them.

- Put the bedrooms as far away from the electrical fuse board as possible.

- Keep human occupied areas away from the electrical fuse board.

- Minimal electric wiring in the home.

- Avoid running electrical cables near to bedroom areas.

- Avoid running cables under floors where children may sit or crawl on the floor. It is better to run them next to the walls.

- No electrical ground rods installed near to the home.

- Install all high current devices as close to the electrical fuse board as possible. This includes electric water heaters, electric cookers, microwave ovens, electric washers, electric dryers, and so on.

- Install all dirty electricity producing products as close to the electrical fuse board as possible. This includes computers, computer networks, televisions, and so on.

- Consider using a dedicated circuit breaker, electrical cable and socket for each noisy electrical product that is on the electrical system.

- Consider installing filters onto dirty electrical circuits.

- Consider using steel conduits for cables on dirty electrical circuits.

- Use photocell smoke alarms.

- Use insulated flooring products to prevent contact with stray voltage that may be in the ground.

- Use plastic plumbing that is kept far away from electrical cables.

- Use products in the home that have a linear current draw, like filament lights.

- Only one electrical outlet in each room unless more are needed, such as in the kitchen.

- Do not run wiring in areas where people may be sleeping near to them.

- Install demand switches that allow you to easily turn off room circuits from within the home.

- Turn off circuits that are not in use at the fuse board.

- Use wood fuel burners for winter heating.

- Avoid living in areas that need to be air conditioned.

- Use gas or wood for cooking and water heating.

- Supplement the water heating with a solar water heater.

- Use "full spectrum" window products. These are generally acrylic instead of glass.

- Make sure that the home has air vents installed in it for fresh air to circulate in from outdoors.

- Use paints that are natural in color and are matte.

- Use outside window coverings instead of inside window coverings. They are far more effective at heat retention in winter and reducing solar heat gain in summer.

- Have a south facing conservatory that is in full winter sunlight in order to provide solar heating for the home in wintertime.

- Do not use metal in the construction, such as a metal roof, metal siding, metal studs, radiant barrier aluminum foil insulation, and so on.

- Use a water catchment system that is sufficiently large enough to hold at least one years supply of water underground. Make sure that it has stone inside it for mineralization of the water.

- Use a cesspool or septic tank for sewage and keep it well away from the electrical ground rods.

- Have a large garden with a growing area for food.

- Use naturally rough materials for paving, such as stone.

- Center the lifestyle around the outdoors with patio's, shade, a court yard for use in breezy days, and outdoor cooking areas.

- Construct your home in an environment that is conducive to living self sufficiently with fertile soil and natural sources of water close by.

The next diagram demonstrates some of these considerations.

"As we live and as we are, Simplicity - with a capital "S" - is difficult to comprehend nowadays. We are no longer truly simple. We no longer live in simple terms or places. Life is a more complex struggle now. It is now valiant to be simple: a courageous thing to even want to be simple. It is a spiritual thing to comprehend what simplicity means."

Frank Lloyd Wright

Healthy Home Design

● Ground rods

Keep this area free of people. Plant trees and shrubs here.

Electricity use should be kept to one side of the home. The bedrooms and bathrooms should be kept far away from the ground rods, fuse board and meter for good health.

Fuse board and meter

Alarm and network

Washer and dryer

Garage

Bedroom

Bath

Bedroom

Keep this area free of people. Plant trees and shrubs here.

Cooker

Kitchen

Refrigerator

Electronics room

TV

Computer

Family room

Master bedroom and bath

Keep this area free of people. Plant trees and shrubs here.

Minimal Electrification

Radiation Sickness

The human is very sensitive to radiation and it is easy to find yourself in the incorrect radiation environment. Factors that feed into radiation sickness are:

- Lack of an annual radiation detoxification cycle.
- The multiple-Sun effect.
- Unnaturally high solar radiation environments.
- Living near to the poles.
- Living in a polluted area, such as a large city.
- Water reflections.
- Snow reflections.
- Exposure to the electrical system.
- Exposure to stray voltage/current/frequency.
- Use of anti-static devices (ASD).
- Exposure to dirty electricity.
- Exposure to products with high amounts of electromagnetic radiation emissions.
- Exposure to transmitter systems.
- The use of wireless products.
- Satellite electromagnetic radiation.
- Contact with metals.
- Sleeping on a metal coil mattress.
- Exposure to moonlight.

- Exposure to sunlight.

- Exposure to artificial lighting products.

- Living at high altitudes.

- Working at high altitudes.

- Exposure to certain types of reflected light.

- Lack of a natural environment with trees and plants.

- Fossil fuel emissions into the atmosphere.

- Water vapor emissions into the atmosphere.

- Industrial emissions into the atmosphere.

- Heat emissions into the atmosphere.

- Human genetics.

- Human skin color.

- Human eye color.

- Human hair color.

- Human clothing.

- The glass in your home, workplace and transportation systems.

- The amount of time that you spend next to a window.

- The construction type of your home and office.

- Your commute to work.

- The transportation systems that you use.

- Make-up.

- Lipstick.

- Painted nails.

- Sunscreen.
- Sunglasses, glasses, and contact lenses.

It is very easy to find yourself in an incorrect radiation state and you will start to get ill if you are not aware of it. The human body appears to only be able to sense just a small amount of the radiation types that contribute to the electromagnetic radiation spectrum.

Regarding environments with high amounts of pollution, you must remember that the human is the bottom dwelling species of a gas ocean. In that ocean the birds and the bees are the fish. The trees are the coral. If you continually pollute that ocean, then you should expect everything to die off. This is exactly what happens when you significantly affect the electromagnetic radiation transmission through air with pollution!

When choosing a home, you should ensure that it is in a green rural environment with few sources of pollution for the best of health.

Track your radiation exposures and learn to stay in the correct radiation environments. Correct daily outdoor solar radiation exposure is extremely important in human health, especially so in the young.

The human body is like a bucket that is constantly filling up with toxins. If the toxic exposures are too high, then those toxins will start to overwhelm the human body. If the toxin level rises quickly, you will get very sick and may go on to develop disease in a short period of time. If the toxin level is rising slowly, then you will slowly get sick and may go on to develop disease over a much longer time period.

Generally, this time period will be years, or even decades. When you examine the human death statistics, you see the the death rate starts rising significantly after the age of thirty and this is when most people start reporting health problems. It appears that many people have become really toxic by the age of thirty!

The only known way to empty out the toxins from the human body is to detoxify.

The human "Toxic Bucket" is shown on the next page.

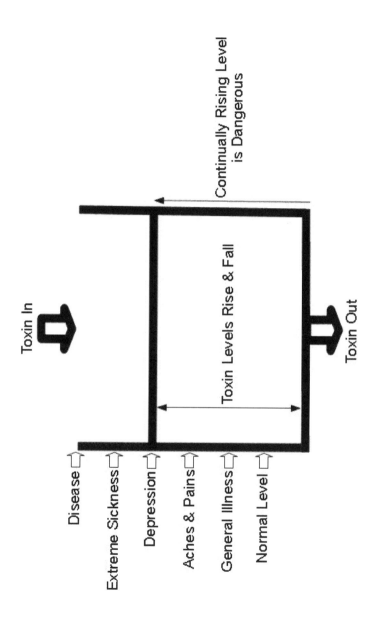

When developing this book, it became apparent that there is a profession that appears to be suffering from radiation sickness and they do not seem to be aware of it. That profession is the police! It is currently documented as "Angry Aggression Theory" and it appears to have the following sources:

- Flashing strobe lights.

- Electromagnetic pulses from strobe lights.

- EMI from their computer systems.

- Artificial light from their computer systems.

- Radio and microwave exposure from their communication devices.

- Cell phone tower and communications tower exposures.

- EMI from electronic weapons.

- EMI from their cars.

- EMI from extended time driving close to high voltage power lines.

- Incorrect daily sunlight exposure.

- Exposure to heavily filtered sunlight.

- Extended exposure to artificial lights.

- Exposure to RADAR and LASER systems.

- Shift work.

"It is my assessment that most police officers who spend their days driving around USA cities will have some level of radiation sickness and this is concerning!"

Steven Magee

Radiation Detoxification

Can you detoxify from radiation? Yes you can! The radiation detoxification can be very painful and extended. It may take several months to go through the first detoxification, and it will vary with the individual and how polluted they are. You should be under medical guidance and supervision if you choose to do this.

Here are the steps that I developed for the radiation detoxification:

- Switch off all but essential electrical circuits at the fuse board.

- Switch off all but essential electrical, electronic and wireless items in your home.

- Change all electric lighting to filament light bulbs.

- Artificial lighting should be minimal and just sufficient for the task.

- Cover all windows with window coverings.

- Your home lighting level should be very low both in the day and the night.

- Do not spend time near the windows.

- Stay covered up with clothing when indoors so that you do not absorb light.

- Keep skin exposure to outdoor light minimal by covering up as much as possible when outside.

- Use dark, neutral density sunglasses and wide brimmed hats when outside.

- Do not use sunscreen, make-up, lipstick, or have painted nails.

- Eat fresh organic food.

- Drink mineral water.

- Go to bed at sunset and wake up at sunrise.

The detoxification can be severe in the first month with flu-like symptoms as you withdraw from natural radiation and artificial radiation exposures.

Fatigue follows for a few months and this can be severe. It gradually gets better the longer you are detoxing. I would recommend that you detoxify for no more than three months at a time. If you detoxify for too long you may go into vitamin D and B12 deficiency, and extreme fatigue may appear. You will know when you are in sunlight deficiency as you will start to get headaches that match the changing levels of sunlight exposure. If you get to this point, then it is time to stop detoxing and to slowly return to sunlight exposure.

Once detoxing is completed, gradually increase your solar radiation exposure to a few hours per day in the shade of trees over several weeks. Obtaining solar radiation in the shade of trees appears to be important in human health due to the modification of solar radiation that takes place in the tree canopy.

The human mind and body can go into solar radiation overload if you spend too much time outdoors and you will need to figure out where the correct solar radiation exposure time is for you by experimentation. Your pain system will let you know if you get too much exposure to solar radiation.

The good news is that after detoxing from radiation exposure, you should feel like a young person again and be free from aches and pains. It is worth the trouble to move into good health.

After the first detoxification, you should detoxify in the middle of winter for forty days and nights each year. The detoxification appears necessary for good human health. After you are detoxed, you will start to realize exactly how much pollution you are being exposed to, as you will feel the effects of it.

Exposure to electromagnetic fields is one of the things that will become very noticeable to you. You will feel like you are allergic to it, due to the reactions that your mind and body will have to it.

This leads me to the conclusion that the reason why people are allergic to pollen is that they have withdrawn too much from nature. The same thing happens with the Sun if you avoid it, you will become "allergic" to it! The only way to start to feel good around things that you are "allergic" to is to continually expose yourself to it so that your body becomes used to the presence of it. It is the same for electromagnetic radiation. Unfortunately, unlike pollen and sunlight, man-made electromagnetic radiation is likely to do long-term damage to your health!

Expanded information on radiation sickness and the radiation detoxification process can be found in the book "Toxic Light".

"The radiation detoxification process exists in nature. It is called: Hibernation."

Steven Magee

Human Safety

In the USA there are a number of safety agencies that have responsibility for human safety in the areas that this book goes into. These are:

- Underwriters Laboratories (UL).

- Federal Communications Commission (FCC).

- Occupational Safety & Health Administration (OSHA).

- Centers for Disease Control and Prevention (CDC).

The Underwriters Laboratories (UL) certification is a product testing standard to ensure that the product meets the minimum criteria for reliable operation, electrocution risks and fire safety.

The FCC certification is for electromagnetic interference with other pieces of equipment. The FCC marking is not a human health standard and the FCC is well aware that all electrical, electronic and wireless equipment is emitting many types of electromagnetic interference fields.

The CDC, OSHA and the FCC are well aware that many researchers have found extensive biological growth defects in plants and animals, and extensive behavioral changes in the human in these man-made electromagnetic radiation fields.

Regarding the FCC and OSHA, I communicated with them prior to writing this book to obtain their historical statistics on the amount of complaints they receive per year and the amount of complaints that they uphold each year. This is one of my emails to the FCC:

Dear Robert,

I have not heard back from you regarding the information below. I am getting ready to copyright my next book and I am after this information from the FCC:

"I am also after a list of the number of complaints that the FCC receives and the number of complaints that the FCC actually upholds each year. I am after the historical data and I would appreciate the public web page that shows this information. If the public web page is not available, then a list of the historical information would be useful that shows the data since the FCC was formed through to now.

In absence of the FCC providing this information to me I will assume a value of 'almost zero percent of complaints to the FCC are ever upheld' for my books. This is in line with my research on the FCC."

Could you also acknowledge the receipt of this information:

"Dear Julius Genachowski,

I would like to formally report these problems to the FCC for investigation:

- *Anti-static devices are causing electrical poisoning to occur in people who use them daily when the electrical grounding system is bad.*

- *"Stray voltage" in the human environment appears to be making large numbers of people ill and may be inducing cancer into them.*

- *My research into electromagnetic interference (EMI) and its effects on human health are matching the same findings as Dr. John Nash Ott reported in his books and films on the subject.*

- *Found that people who live near street lights have a higher risk of premature death and illness due to a combination of the radio wave fields that they emit and the relatively monochromatic spectrum of light.*

- *That the electrical distribution system is in the process of turning into an unlicensed broadband radio transmitter due to high penetrations of electronic generation and electronic loads that create harmonics. This will cause radio wave sickness (RWS) and electromagnetic hypersensitivity (EHS) to occur in many people.*

- *Found that the human mating and fertility cycles are triggered by exposure to electromagnetic interference from electrical storms, and that the modern human is unnaturally being stimulated by daily electromagnetic interference (EMI) exposure. Over exposure to EMI causes aggression and fatigue to occur.*

- *Found that many electronic products are emitting large amounts of EMI and radio waves that are easily detectable with an AM radio tuned to static.*

- *Found that many electrical utility power poles and lines are emitting large amounts of radio waves into the human environment. They are unlicensed broadband radio transmitters.*

- *EMI exposure appears to cause the following issues in humans: increased sexual desire, aggression, fatigue, mental illness, depression, illness and cancer.*

- *Widespread radiation sickness in the modern human environment from the effects of unnatural solar radiation, man-made radiation, and electromagnetic interference.*

I have attached my resume for you to see and I look forward to hearing from you soon."

I do regard silence as a form of lying and I hope that you do not continue to meet my requests for basic information in this way. I have attached my latest resume for you to see that lists my latest discoveries regarding electromagnetic radiation and human health and I look forward to hearing from you within the next week.

Yours sincerely,

Steven Magee

The FCC did eventually supply an internet link, but did not supply the requested information. The link that they supplied is here:

http://www.fcc.gov/encyclopedia/quarterly-reports-consumer-inquiries-and-complaints

When I pointed out to them that it did not match my request, they responded:

This seems the type of information that the Freedom of Information Act (FOIA) was designed to disclose. Instructions for filing a FOIA request are available at:

http://www.fcc.gov/guides/how-file-foia-request

Be aware, however, that the FOIA does not require an agency to create new information. So, if there are no records concerning numbers of complaints being "upheld," then there is nothing to be produced.

Time ran out during working on the first edition of this book for the dialog to go to the conclusion of a FOIA request. And quite frankly, I had lost interest in obtaining the information as they appear to not want to supply it. One can only wonder what information that they would eventually supply when harassed for it, as it is very easy to modify data.

Regarding the OSHA numbers, despite two separate requests to them, no response was generated by them.

My independent research indicates that it is below 5% and may actually be close to zero percent of cases ever upheld.

Many researchers report the government's secrecy in these systems of apparent "public protection". If you are able to obtain these numbers, I would be interested to hear from you.

As can be seen from the above emails, the USA government responds with a combination of silence, misinformation, and not recording certain types of information regarding inconvenient truths. Dr. John Nash Ott extensively documents these types of actions by corporations and government departments that he tried to inform about his important research.

To understand this problem with public protection, you need to take a look at how the government, corporate, and public protection money flows are routed. This is shown on the next page.

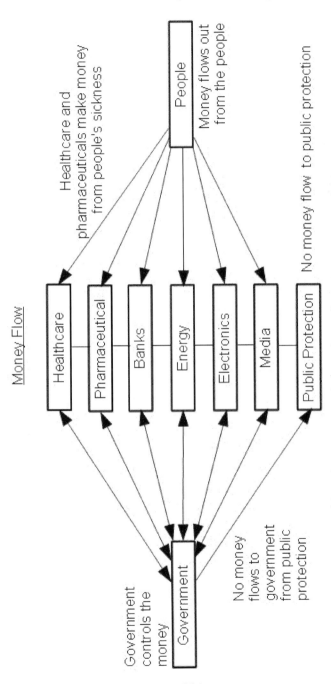

Corporations took control of the government a long time ago through political donations and political lobbying. The corporations are extensively linked together through business organizations, like the Chamber of Commerce and trade associations. As such, political lobbying is organized between the various types of corporations to obtain an outcome that is beneficial to the majority of them.

It is well known that we have had decades of deregulation in the USA and this was driven by corporate lobbying and political donations. Deregulation simply means that the government has extensively cut oversight to the organizations. As such, this leaves many corporations with little to no oversight.

Part of the corporate deregulation process was to extensively remove accountability for health and safety. Keeping workers safe can be an expensive overhead in some industries and the only way to drive down costs in this area is to deregulate the health and safety system. This happened a long time ago in the USA. As such, there are many health and safety laws that the corporations are supposed to comply with, but are no longer enforced.

You would be shocked at how little of the health and safety system is enforced today in the USA. It appears for this reason they will not tell researchers how many complaints they uphold, as it is so few!

The OSHA statement *"You have the right to a safe workplace"* may actually be recorded by future historians as one of the biggest lies ever told to the general population!

This has led to a corporate system that is routinely selling known toxic products to an unsuspecting mass population. And there is absolutely nothing that the workers who are witnessing these unlawful acts can do about it, as the health and safety system was deregulated!

As a result of the willful failure of these government agencies to protect the public health, the modern human can be compared to a zombie today due to the amount of toxins that it has allowed itself to be exposed to. The modern human thinks differently, acts differently, and dies differently to those of the past, prior to the introduction of electricity.

I have no doubts that the CDC, OSHA and the FCC will be remembered as government agencies that willfully failed to protect the general public from fraudulent corporate and government activities. They will probably be recorded in the future historical records as agencies that were formed to give an illusion of protection to the general public.

The human health problems that they have willfully failed to prevent are massive and extend into arthritis, joint disorders, heart attacks, circulation issues, obesity, system deficiencies, system toxicity, fatigue, depression, electrical poisoning, radio wave sickness, microwave sickness, radiation sickness, mental health, childhood development problems, Autism, Attention Deficit Disorder (ADD), aggression, violence, electromagnetic hypersensitivity, and so on.

They did assist the corporations in making massive profits at the expense of the health of the past, current, and future generations of humans. The energy, electronics, pharmaceutical, and healthcare industries are massive in the USA, as is their influence on the USA government. It would appear that protecting corporate profits is far more important than protecting human health in the USA.

My interactions with government agencies regarding safety issues and the discoveries that I made during the course of developing my publications revealed a system that I can only describe as shockingly bad. It is rare to get an acknowledgment of communication. They generally refuse through silence to engage in two way discussions. They enable corporations to willfully break multiple USA laws and avoid prosecution. And above all, they do not seem at all interested in protecting the health and well being of the general public and their offspring.

It is my conclusion that there are far more profits to be made from selling toxic products to sick people than there is in a healthy population. Clearly, to sell toxic products relies on the general public not understanding the toxicity of the products that they purchase. Electricity and the various forms of radiation have been known to be toxic for decades and the government is staying silent about it.

Until that changes, you should ensure that you are aware of the toxicity of electricity and act accordingly if you value your health.

The modern human is shown in the next photograph.

"Nothing strengthens authority so much as silence."
Leonardo da Vinci

Exposure to the various forms of harmful electricity has been turning many people into "zombies" for over a hundred years now.

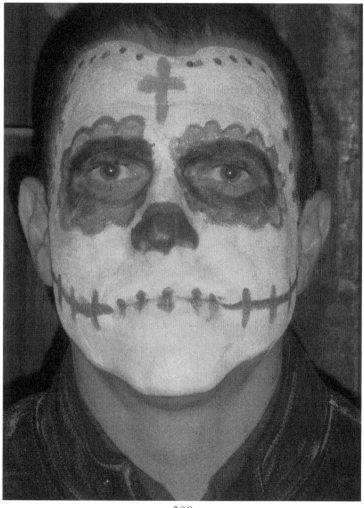

<u>Utility Company Deceit</u>

The electrical utility companies are nice, aren't they? They would not hide the toxicity of electricity for many decades from the general public, would they?

Here is a small excerpt of a large USA utility electricity company contract:

5. In exchange for the consideration set forth in this Agreement, SUBORDINATE waives his right to sue UTILITY for any matter whatsoever, whether known or unknown, for any conduct, acts, omissions, or causes of action arising from the beginning of time up through the Effective Date of this Agreement, except an action to challenge the validity of SUBORDINATE's release of claims under (i) the Age Discrimination in Employment Act of 1967 (ADEA), 29 U.S.C. § 621 et seq. (which statute generally prohibits age discrimination in employment) and/or (ii) the Older Workers Benefit Protection Act (OWBPA), 29 U.S.C. § 621 et seq. (which statute was enacted to, among other things, ensure that individuals over the age of forty who waive their rights under the ADEA do so knowingly and voluntarily). In addition, SUBORDINATE releases UTILITY from all claims which he has or may have from the beginning of time up through the Effective Date of this Agreement, and expressly agrees not to file a lawsuit to assert any such claims. SUBORDINATE also waives his right to recover in any action which may be brought on his behalf by any person or entity, including any governmental agency such as, for example, the Equal Employment Opportunity Commission or the Department of Labor. The foregoing agencies are meant to be illustrative rather than all-inclusive.

6. This General Release ("Release") is a FULL AND FINAL BAR TO ANY CLAIMS which SUBORDINATE has or may have against UTILITY, except SUBORDINATE is not releasing his right to challenge the validity of his release of claims under the ADEA and/or OWBPA. By entering into this Agreement, SUBORDINATE knowingly and voluntarily releases, waives, and forever discharges UTILITY from any and all claims, demands, damages, debts, obligations, promises, covenants, agreements, contracts, actions, suits, or causes of action, of any kind whatsoever, in law or equity, whether known or unknown, disclosed or undisclosed, foreseen or unforeseen, foreseeable or unforeseeable, and any consequences thereof, which he has or may have through the Effective Date of this Agreement, including, but not limited to, any claim(s) under the:

A. Age Discrimination in Employment Act of 1967 (ADEA), 29 U.S.C. § 621 et seq. (which statute generally prohibits age discrimination in employment);

B. Employee Retirement Income Security Act of 1974 (ERISA), 29 U.S.C. § 1001 et seq., including but not limited to Sections 502 and 510 (which statute was enacted to, among other things, help protect an employee's interest in their pension benefits);

C. Americans with Disabilities Act (ADA), 42 U.S.C. § 12101 et seq. (which statute generally prohibits disability discrimination);

D. *Title VII of the Civil Rights Act of 1964, as amended, 42 U.S.C. § 2000e et seq. (which statute generally prohibits discrimination in employment based on race, color, religion, national origin or sex);*

E. *National Labor Relations Act (NLRA), 29 U.S.C. § 151 et seq. (which statute protects certain concerted activity as well as the rights of employees to organize and bargain collectively through representatives with their employer);*

F. *Fair Credit Reporting Act (FCRA), 15 U.S.C. § 1681 et seq. (which statute requires certain disclosures and consent by an individual before a consumer reporting agency may communicate information about the individual to an employer);*

G. *Equal Pay Act (EPA), 29 U.S.C. § 206 (which statute generally prohibits unequal pay for equal work between men and women);*

H. *Older Workers Benefit Protection Act (OWBPA), 29 U.S.C. § 621 et seq. (which statute was enacted to, among other things, ensure that individuals over the age of forty who waive their rights under the ADEA do so knowingly and voluntarily);*

1. *42 U.S.C. § 1981 (which statute generally prohibits race discrimination);*

J. Occupational Safety and Health Act of 1970 (OSHA), 29 U.S.C. § 651 et seq. (which statute is designed to ensure a safe and healthful work environment);

K. Worker Adjustment and Retraining Notification Act (WARN), 29 U.S.C. § 2101 et seq. (which statute requires advance notice to employees before their business establishment is closed);

L. Sarbanes-Oxley Act of 2002 (which statute prohibits, among other things, discrimination against whistleblowing in publicly-traded companies);

M. Family & Medical Leave Act (FMLA), 29 U.S.C. § 2601 et seq. (which statute provides for unpaid leave for eligible employees for certain qualifying events);

N. Any other federal, state, or local civil or human rights law, regulation, or ordinance, including but not limited to the Florida Civil Rights Act of 1992, Broward County Human Rights Act, City of West Palm Beach Equal Opportunity Ordinance (Chapter 34), Palm Beach County Equal Employment Ordinance, and the Miami-Dade County Code (Chapter 1 lA) (all dealing with employment discrimination);

O. Any and all claims/actions which have been or could have been raised under Florida's workers' compensation statute (Chapter 440), including but not limited to any claims/actions under the retaliation section of that statute (Florida Statute § 440.205);

P. Any and all rights and claims under Florida's "Whistleblower" law (Florida Statute § 448.102). SUBORDINATE states that he has not been retaliated against in any personnel action for disclosing or threatening to disclose any activity, policy, or practice of UTILITY which is allegedly in violation of any law, rule, or regulation; or for providing information or testifying about such activity, policy, or practice; or for objecting to or refusing to participate in such activity, policy, or practice;

Q. Claims based upon any UTILITY benefit program or plan of any type in which SUBORDINATE has not yet vested, except as may otherwise be set forth in this Agreement; and/or

R. Any claims of violation of public policy, unpaid wages, breach of contract, negligent or intentional infliction of emotional distress, defamation, assault, battery, false imprisonment, wrongful termination, negligent hiring, retention, or supervision, fraud; misrepresentation; qui tam provisions of any local, state, or federal law; or any other claim of any type, whether based on common law, statute, or otherwise.

The foregoing list is meant to be illustrative rather than all-inclusive. SUBORDINATE IS WAIVING ALL RIGHTS AND CLAIMS (IF ANY) WHICH HE HAS OR MAY HAVE AGAINST UTILITY through the Effective Date of this Agreement, except his right to challenge the validity of his release of claims under the ADEA and/or OWBPA.

Notwithstanding anything to the contrary in this Agreement, SUBORDINATE is not releasing: (i) any rights to any vested benefit under any employee benefit plan, as defined by ERISA; (ii) COBRA continuation coverage, as applicable; (iii) any rights provided in this Agreement; (iv) any rights to challenge the validity of SUBORDINATE's release of claims under the ADEA and/or OWBPA; or (v) any rights or claims which may arise after the Effective Date of this Agreement.

As you can see, it is clearly an illegal document. It appears that in the USA electrical utility industry, employees are stripped of all of their legal and civil rights. What is more concerning is that they are stripping employees of their health and safety rights!

This particular utility runs a very large fleet of nuclear reactors in the USA, in addition to its portfolio of conventional, and renewable wind and solar generation facilities. It has won many awards for its ethical behaviors.

One has to wonder how an unethical company that is breaking many USA laws daily can possibly be winning awards for its ethical behaviors? The answer is simply that this is how corruption works.

Some of the most corrupt companies in the world are actually the ones that you think are the most environmentally friendly. The concept is known as "greenwashing". Wikipedia states:

Greenwashing (a compound word modeled on "whitewash"), or "green sheen", is a form of spin in which green PR or green marketing is deceptively used to promote the perception that an organization's aims and policies are environmentally friendly. Whether it is to increase profits or gain political support, greenwashing may be used to manipulate popular opinion to support otherwise questionable aims.

Greenwashing is a form of propaganda that is used by electrical utility companies to garner public support for their agenda. These same companies are the ones that are staying quiet about the toxicity of their electrical systems.

"Lying through silence" is a feature of the modern world that we now live in.

As can be seen from the contract, the electrical utility companies appear to think that hundreds of years of well developed federal laws, state laws, county laws, city laws, civil rights laws, and health and safety laws do not apply to them. This arrogance is why today we have an electricity system that is poisoning people in very large numbers.

The utility company lawyers have assessed the situation and have decided that these toxic effects take many years to develop in the human mind and body, need specialized knowledge to detect them, and are very difficult to prove in a court of law. So it is far cheaper to pay the few successful lawsuits than it is to make the system safe for the many.

Utility companies have seen the results of toxic electricity many times. It is extensively documented in the book "Electrocution of America" by Russ Allen. This particular book only details one toxic aspect of the electrical system that is called "stray voltage" and the devastating impact it had on both his family and their farm animals. The electrical system has many toxic aspects to it.

When an electrical utility company is threatened with an investigation or lawsuit, it finds a group of long term trusted employees that can willfully lie under oath. They will generally be older managers of groups. It then sits them in a room with the army of highly paid electrical utility lawyers and they draw up a battle plan on how to make the person(s) look so bad and incompetent that they will lose the case. Generally, the majority of this information is untrue. They know it is untrue and they are completely okay with this. Lying under oath is a normal part of business for them. You will generally not find the newer employees in the company engaging in the practice. It is something that comes with exposure to the electrical utility company's lack of ethics. These "expert" electrical utility company witnesses generally get excellent annual bonuses and earn very large salaries. To get to the top in the electrical utility field, you need to have "Pinocchio" ethics!

Russ Allen documents a blatant disregard for his family's health and that of his farm animals. He eventually had to take his electrical utility company to court and won the case. He was awarded $1,750,000 USA dollars. In 2013 a USA family was awarded four million dollars for the harm electromagnetic fields and stray voltage caused them that their utility company refused to fix. They ended up with nerve damage.

I can confirm that the behaviors that Russ Allen documents in his book have also been demonstrated by my own utility company.

When researching anti-static devices (ASD), I found that my tiled floors are electrified in my home with 60 Hz AC voltage! I reported it to the utility company who closed the case without performing a single measurement at my home that would demonstrate the presence of stray voltage. When I invited them into my home to witness my measurements, they stayed silent. The voltage is still there today!

This was my response to them closing the investigation:

Hi Jeremiah,

I have not heard from you in over a week with regards to attending my property to witness my measurements of "Stray Voltage" that I have traced to TEP's floating neutral system. At this point I am assuming that both TEP and yourself are willfully violating the laws of the United States. Both the staff at TEP and yourself may end up in jail if it is later proven that you were engaging in willful criminal negligence.

You are electrifying the sidewalks, the tiled flooring of the homes, and the gardens of the homes. In some homes in the area you are likely electrifying the swimming pools and water systems of these homes. I have yet to see TEP actually try to measure for stray voltage effects on your neutral system. You have installed two loggers that I witnessed the installation of and no reference to a non-electrified ground connection was made.

As a Chartered Electrical Engineer, it has been frustrating to witness such incompetence. It is clear that TEP is completely okay with electrifying the side walks and the human environment with no regard to the human health consequences that such actions may have. Clearly, to know that you are electrifying a residential area that has developing babies and children in it and not to fix the known health hazard that this presents is, in my opinion, an act of criminal negligence.

Again, the problem that I have requested for you to diagnose and fix is one of "stray voltage" that is originating at your neutral. The possible causes for this are:

- *Insufficiently sized neutral cables*
- *Corroded neutral cables*
- *Loose neutral cables*
- *The ground in the area is insufficiently conductive for use as an electrical ground system*
- *An insulation fault on your live conductor that is electrifying the ground in the area*

The fault is still present at my home and it originates at your neutral system. Please fix it.

Yours sincerely,

Steven Magee

I reported it to the Arizona Corporate Commission (ACC) who are the government agency that regulate them and they have never acknowledged nor responded to my complaint.

There are some movies that document energy company and government regulator problems:

- "Silkwood" is a 1983 American drama film directed by Mike Nichols. The screenplay by Nora Ephron and Alice Arlen was inspired by the life of Karen Silkwood, a labor union activist who died in a suspicious car accident while investigating alleged wrongdoing at the Kerr-McGee plutonium plant where she worked.

- "Erin Brockovich" is a 2000 biographical film directed by Steven Soderbergh. The film is a dramatization of the true story of Erin Brockovich, portrayed by Julia Roberts, who fought against the US West Coast energy corporation Pacific Gas and Electric Company (PG&E).

- "Gasland" and "Gasland Part 2" are American documentaries written and directed by Josh Fox. The films focus on communities in the United States impacted by natural gas drilling and, specifically, a method of horizontal drilling into shale formations known as slickwater fracking.

- "Take Back Your Power" is an eye-opening documentary which investigates the "smart" meter program currently being implemented worldwide by most of the major utility companies. These devices are being installed often without the consent – and sometimes against the protests – of property owners. The film uncovers alarming issues about health, privacy, property rights, corporate fraud, and vulnerability issues inherent in the "smart" grid.

This leads me to conclude this chapter with the following question:

"What is government if words have no meaning?"

RWS & EHS

Radio Wave Sickness (RWS) and Electromagnetic Hypersensitivity (EHS) are rapidly accelerating plagues in modern society. Sweden appears to be the only country that currently recognizes the conditions. In Sweden approximately 300,000 people are registered as having EHS. Sweden has a population of 9,555,893 as reported in the 2012 census. This equates to 3.12 percent of the population, or 1 in 32 people, that is aware that it is being affected by unnatural radiation exposures which include electrical, electronic and wireless systems. Elizabeth Kelley, electromagneticsafety.org, reports that:

Since the early 1990s, health practitioners world-wide have seen a rapid increase in the number of people who report a cluster of neurological symptoms that is called electromagnetic hypersensitivity. EHS symptoms commonly include headache, sleep problems, poor memory and concentration, depression, anxiety, changes in heart rate and, skin burning sensations. These symptoms are being reported mainly by people who live in the developed world where there has been rapid human adaptation to wireless digital technologies over the past two decades.

In 2005, the World Health Organization published Fact Sheet No 296 entitled Electromagnetic Hypersensitivity: "Well controlled and conducted double-blind studies have shown that symptoms were not correlated with EMF exposure... The symptoms are certainly real and can vary widely in their severity... Further, EHS is not a medical diagnosis, nor is it clear that it represents a single medical problem."

Dr. Olle Johannsson, a Swedish neuroscientist, reports that in Sweden electrohypersensitivity (EHS) is an officially fully recognized functional impairment and those who have this condition are eligible for government services and accommodations. Recent studies show that over 5% of Swedish men and women report a variety of symptoms when exposed to electromagnetic field (EMF) sources.

Dr. Magda Havas, a professor of environmental science at Trent University in Ontario Canada, states that EHS studies with negative results can have major biases. "The researchers assumed that reactions to EMFs are immediate, while there is often a delay between exposure and response. People are not switches that can be turned on and off. These studies incorrectly insinuate that, if you can't feel anything, it can't harm you. We know very well that we can't detect the taste of arsenic, lead, DDT nor asbestos, but they are all toxic."

European medical doctors are estimating that, by 2017, 50% of the world's population will be affected by mild to severe EHS symptoms.

The problem with RWS and EHS in the USA is that it is commonly misdiagnosed as another condition. The USA has become addicted to wireless communications technologies and electrical and electronic products, so the rates are likely comparable to Sweden. The recent adoption of Smart/AMR/AMI radiation transmitting utility meters in many USA cities has probably significantly increased the number of people who have RWS and EHS, but are currently incorrectly diagnosed.

This is unfortunate, as it is well known today that RWS and EHS is easily preventable. All you have to do is remove the sources of man-made electromagnetic interference. I find it very concerning that the USA government simply ignores people who are trying to restore their environment back to natural radiation levels in an effort to clear up their RWS and EHS symptoms. It appears to be rare for the Federal Communications Commission (FCC) to enforce rule 15 that relates to harmful electromagnetic interference. Indeed, I recently put rule 15 to the test and notified the FCC that the gas company was causing biologically harmful interference at my home. They simply ignored my request for them to notify the gas company to remove their biologically harmful transmitting meters from the area around my home.

The FCC have established one of the most lax electromagnetic radiation standards in the world. At 61 volts per meter (V/m) for 1800 MHz public exposure, the permissible radiation emissions are higher than most other countries in the world. For contrast, 0.06 V/m is the recommendation in Salzburg, Austria, which makes the USA standard 1017 times higher! The reason for this ridiculously high standard in the USA is obvious when you look at the military. The most technologically advanced military in the world has been developing wireless warfare for decades. If the FCC was to lower the standards, then they would effectively render some parts of the military arsenal as obsolete.

This same military force who became aware of what RWS and EHS was during the development of RADAR in the 1930's and 1940's appears to have been denying the condition exists from the 1950's onwards! Instead, the opposite happened and electrical, electronic and wireless products were heavily marketed to the masses, while the military who were supposed to protect them from biological harm simply stayed silent.

When you look into how electrical, electronic and wireless products are approved for sale in the USA, you find that no laboratory animals are used to assess their safety. Instead, electronic meters make measurements and something that resembles Jello is used to assess if the devices can heat it. If the meter readings are within specification and the Jello is not substantially heated, then the product is approved for sale.

The reality is that if these devices were tested on animals and plants, then many of them would fail the tests! As Dr. John Nash Ott discovered in his research that he conducted from the 1950's to the 1980's, many electrical and electronic products change the behaviors of animals and can make them sick, and some of them go on to die premature deaths. He also found that if you subjected an animal to biologically harmful electromagnetic radiation and made it sick, that you could return it to a healthy state simply by removing the harmful exposures. This is exactly what people are reporting who have RWS and EHS!

Dr. John Nash Ott performed many plant experiments with electromagnetic radiation and he found that plants would react to many common electrical and electronic products.

Growth deformities were observed in many of his experiments. I have been able to reproduce much of his work regarding plants and I can tell you that his findings are easily repeatable.

Many government agencies are aware of not only Dr. John Nash Ott's work, but also of the work done by many other researchers. Indeed, I have mailed many dozens of copies of my books to government agencies. It is rare to get a response and when I do get one, it is typically an acknowledgment that they received the book. It is a similar story at the universities.

People are now reporting curing Autism by electromagnetically shielding the child's bedroom. This is consistent with Autism being an electromagnetic disease and may indeed be easily preventable. The Autism rates have been closely following the rise in cell phone towers and cell phones in the USA over the past decade. Transmitting Smart/AMR/AMI utility meters should be expected to increase the Autism rates, as they create a high powered antenna park at the home that is constantly transmitting pulsed radiation for approximately one mile in residential areas. Pulsed radiation is the most biologically harmful form of radiation transmission.

Electromagnetic shielding is a common response to the problem of electromagnetic radiation. You need to be very careful with shielding, as you can make the problem worse. I have been growing plants in Faraday cages and I have seen extensive growth problems occurring. Some people are inadvertently living in electromagnetically shielded homes and this may occur

through the use of metal roofs, metal siding, foil radiant barriers, and insulation and windows that have electromagnetic shielding properties. Long term sickness may occur when living in such a home that may be accompanied by childhood development problems. You should not electromagnetically shield homes and workplaces as you may create radiation deficiency conditions in the inhabitants.

It is one of the dilemmas with RWS and EHS, to get sick from living in an unnaturally high radiation environment, or to get sick from an electromagnetically screened radiation deficient environment. Either way, many humans will eventually get sick! Even pregnant mothers are electromagnetically shielding their unborn babies with a product called "Belly Armor". This action may eventually make them sick from radiation deficiency problems, similar to what astronauts show that live on the International Space Station for many months. The only known effective solution to RWS and EHS is to return your radiation environment back to natural levels.

The human environment is no longer natural and this increasing of the radiation environment should be expected to rapidly accelerate human evolution into an electromagnetically hardened animal. Unfortunately, many humans will die after many years of easily preventable illness and disease during this period that we are currently in.

The precursor to disease are strange health conditions showing up. Radio Wave Sickness is well categorized today and the top reported radio wave sickness symptoms in order of frequency are:

1. *Fatigue.*

2. *Sleep disturbance.*

3. *Headaches.*

4. *Feeling of discomfort.*

5. *Difficulty in concentrating.*

6. *Depression.*

7. *Memory loss.*

8. *Visual disruptions.*

9. *Irritability.*

10. *Hearing disruptions.*

11. *Skin problems.*

12. *Cardiovascular.*

13. *Dizziness.*

14. *Loss of appetite.*

15. *Movement difficulties*

16. *Nausea.*

Source: Symptoms experiences by people in the vicinity of cellular phone base station, Santini 2001, La Presse Medical.

Indeed, it is well known today that the sickness rates increase within a quarter mile of a cell phone tower. The closer you are to it, the more likely it is for you to be sick. The utilities installing Smart/AMR/AMI meters at your home and in your neighborhood is comparable to turning your home into an antenna park.

When looking back in history we can find documented illnesses that are comparable to RWS and EHS:

- 1829 - Neurasthenia (Also called Americanitis or Nervosism): As a psychopathological term, neurasthenia was used by George Miller Beard in 1869 to denote a condition with symptoms of fatigue, anxiety, headache, neuralgia and depressed mood. This condition showed up in the population during the construction of the railroads and the telegraph that shorted out the semiconductor properties of the natural ground and created man-made electromagnetic interference. It was associated with upper class people and with professionals working in sedentary occupations.

- Mid 1800's - Female Hysteria: Women considered to be suffering from it exhibited a wide array of symptoms including faintness, nervousness, sexual desire, insomnia, fluid retention, heaviness in abdomen, muscle spasm, shortness of breath, irritability, loss of appetite for food or sex, and "a tendency to cause trouble". The women at the time were wearing steel hoop skirts and steel crinolines that would have been acting as antenna systems and electromagnetic shields to electromagetic energy.

- Early 1900's - Shenjing Shuairuo: Chinese equivalent of Neurasthenia. The condition is associated with a collection of symptoms including amnesia, dizziness, fatigue, gastrointestinal disorders, headaches, pain in joints and muscles, poor concentration and sexual dysfunction. This appears to match with the adoption of electricity into the cities.

Full Size Female Hysteria Metal Skirt Experiment

The Palo Verde tree is wearing a steel hoop skirt to see if it will show abnormal growth patterns. The rings are currently insulated from each other and will be connected together the following year with steel wire to turn it into a crinoline.

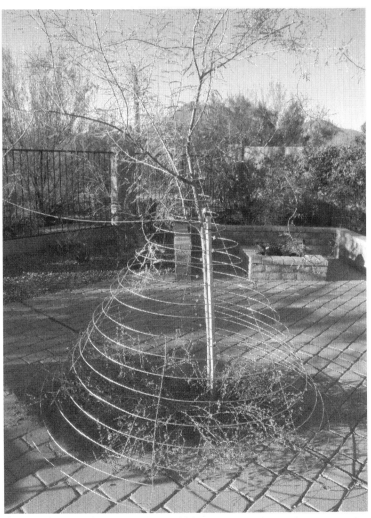

If you are currently experiencing the symptoms of RWS and EHS, I would recommend that you work on changing the electrical characteristics of your body. Changing the electrical characteristics of the human body can help to alleviate the symptoms of RWS and EHS. There are several proven ways to do this:

- Change your fluid intake.

- Change your diet.

- Exercise.

- Sweat.

- Go into a hot or cold environment.

- Build up muscle mass in every part of the body.

- Reduce or increase your weight.

- Submerge the body in water, such as a bath or swimming pool.

- Have no metal near to nor in contact with the body.

- Have no electrical nor electronic products near to nor in contact with the body.

- Do not wear a battery powered watch.

- Wear clothes made out of natural materials.

- Make sure that you are not wearing shoes that create static.

- Wear conductive shoes or walk barefoot in areas that have no stray voltage problems.

- Sleep on the ground on a thin insulated mat to couple into it through capacitance. Make sure that there are no electrical cables in the ground.

- **Sleep directly in contact with the ground in areas that do not have stray voltage/current/frequency problems.**

- **Remove metal from the body, such as dental fillings, dental implants and dental bridges.**

Regarding removing implants from the body, you should regard this as a last resort. There are many steps that you can take that may alleviate your symptoms and they are far easier than having implants removed. While metal implants are known for their ability to induce RWS and EHS into the human, you may be able to clear up the conditions without having to remove these. Of course, if you do not have metal implants, then you should ensure that you do not get them in the future.

You should also pay attention to your pets. Looks for signs of RWS and EHS in them, as they can be an early warning sign that your environmental conditions are unnatural. I remember my grandfathers male dog always being sexually excited and aggressive. It would occasionally go crazy and run at full speed around the home for no reason. I suspect that he was walking the dog in areas that had stray voltage, stray currents and stray frequencies in them. My grandfather went on to die of Dementia which is associated with stray voltage, stray current and stray frequency exposure. He was probably being exposed to the same energies as the dog through the conductive dog leash and his leather soled shoes.

I have every expectation that in time, Dr. John Nash Ott will be recognized as the man who could have prevented the Autism epidemic and many other conditions as well!

Dr. John Nash Ott was working in areas of "Inconvenient Truths" and the people who he was trying to inform about his valuable work simply ignored him, as it would have greatly affected their business model to acknowledge his work. Simply profits before people.

The modern human is derelict in its duty to the next generation who cannot protect themselves from harm. This madness must be stopped. The modern human is displaying an apathy in the above areas that is leading to great levels of easily preventable sickness occurring in the current adult generations and retardation appearing in large numbers in the next generation. Indeed, experts in the field of Autism are indicating that at the currently accelerating levels, in fifteen years every USA child will have an Autism diagnosis!

"Radio Wave Sickness and Electromagnetic Hypersensitivity are easily preventable and one can only wonder how much longer the insanity of modern governments is going to be allowed to continue in this area."

Steven Magee

My Experiences

I started to play around with electricity when I was thirteen years old. Around that time I got my first home computer system which was to spark an interest in electricity and electronics. I left school at sixteen and became an apprentice electrician at the city center university research and teaching hospital. I worked in the electrical group for ten years and I have to say that I noticed people changing during that time.

I had noticed that some of the electricians had made the electrical rooms into workshops and they spent most of their day in them. In particular, there were two electricians who used to take their breaks in these rooms and sleep against the high powered switchgear. They had very strange personalities!

In 1987 the hospital was in the process of switching over from conventional florescent lighting to electronic florescent lighting and installing computer systems for the medical records. There were robots in the sterile areas, ultrasonic baths, high frequency induction furnaces in the laboratories, RADAR operated automatic doors, and so on. I was working with many modern devices and no one ever warned me about the toxicity of these. In fact, no one ever told me about effects such as stray voltage/current/frequency, electromagnetic radiation health problems, harmonic energy making electromagnetic fields on cables get very large, pulsating magnetic fields affecting the brain, electrical and electronic field emissions and to stay out of them.

I would regularly walk through the hospital underground distribution system corridors and be inches from 6,600 volt AC electricity power cables and florescent lights. We would smash up the numerous florescent tubes that we would change every week, releasing toxic clouds of mercury contaminated white phosphor dust. Today, I can only imagine what these things must have been doing to my biological health!

The thing about working in a hospital is that you get to meet a lot of people who are sick and dying. I would have many conversations with these people over the years. The consistent thing that they would repeatedly say to me was that they could not understand how they had become ill. It was always a mystery to them.

It is interesting that in 1987 Dr. John Nash Ott had actually published all of his research into electromagnetic radiation:

- My Ivory Cellar; [The Story of Time-Lapse Photography]. 1958.

- Health and Light: The Extraordinary Study That Shows How Light Affects Your Health and Emotional Well Being. 1973.

- Exploring the Spectrum: The Effects of Natural and Artificial Light on Living Organisms. 1975.

- Light, Radiation, and You: How to Stay Healthy. 1982.

- Color and Light: Their Effects on Plants, Animals and People. 1987.

Dr. John Nash Ott had discovered by 1987 that glass, artificial light sources, electricity and electronic systems were having extensive detrimental effects on plants, animals and humans. No one at the hospital was talking about it. The hospital had 1,000 beds, an animal research facility, a university research facility, a nursing teaching center, a doctors teaching center, a dental teaching center and on site residence buildings to house all of the students. It was a huge university campus! One can only wonder why no one was talking about the toxicity of light, electricity, electronic systems and wireless radiation.

As well as my day job, I would go to college and university one day and one night per week. I obtained an Ordinary National Certificate, Higher National Certificate, Higher National Diploma, and a Bachelors with Honors in Electrical and Electronic Engineering. I can tell you that in ten years of studying electricity and electronics, not one mention was ever made of the toxicity of electricity.

Dr. John Nash Ott authored his last publication in 1987. I graduated in 1996, some nine years later. His work was never mentioned in any of my classes nor text books on the subject. No teachings were given to me about the toxicity of electricity. Harmonics was taught, but only for its effects on electrical equipment, not human health. No mention was ever made about the very large electromagnetic fields that it puts onto cables and equipment.

One of the things that I remember as an apprentice was that when I started at the hospital, I was extremely fatigued for the first few months of working there. The mechanical apprentice who started at the same time as me was reporting the same thing. Today, I know that effect to be the body adjusting to toxic environmental conditions.

Both the mechanical apprentice and myself were from rural areas outside of the city. Working at a highly industrialized facility in the city center was an alien environment for us. In addition to the variety of modern equipment that the hospital had, it had a large number of telecommunications radio frequency transmission antenna systems on the roof. Today it is known that these systems are harmful to the human at close proximity. We were constantly working near the antenna systems with no precautions.

I had found the people in the facilities team to be mostly pleasant, but a little strange too. I had also noticed personalities changing during the ten years that I worked in this group, my own personality was also changing. In particular, I do remember one of the members of the electrical team being exceptionally friendly and very smart and he actually became the opposite, unfriendly and mean during the time I knew him. The adoption of electronics and computer systems into the hospital had become rampant during that time period. This particular person had a number of metal implants that today we know to be incompatible with exposure to the various forms of electricity.

I had noticed that my face was constantly flushing and that my memory was having issues. Forgetfulness was

quite normal during my time there and I was always tired. My mating cycle was frequently being triggered and I thought it was normal. I had never known any different.

In 1996 I changed my position and started working with dialysis machines. These were highly complex computer controlled machines that were filled with the latest electrical and electronic products. The joke in the group was that everyone who joined the team got divorced shortly afterwords! Little did they know that it was the electromagnetic interference emissions from the machines that was probably causing it.

I had noticed my health significantly degrading in my late twenties after joining this group. General aches and pains, feeling lethargic, nosebleeds, mouth ulcers, lung pains, gums bleeding after brushing my teeth and being extremely tired in the mornings had become normal. Getting up in the mornings was always difficult. Working on my home during the weekends was a problem due to the low energy levels. I later realized that part of this may have been coming from drinking reverse osmosis water. The dialysis team was making its tea and coffee with the same reverse osmosis water that the machines used! Reverse osmosis water is highly processed water that is extremely mineral deficient!

It was the first position that had issued me with a laptop computer system, anti-static strap and pager. I remember seeing the doctor about recurring chapped lips that had shown up in this position and they told me it was normal. I now know that it was exposure to the artificial light from the laptop computer that was causing this. The pager was constantly clipped to my belt and would work throughout the region, so I know that I was in extensive unnatural radio fields that communicated with it. I would have the pager with me, even when I slept. I do wonder if the early pager systems had harmful biological emissions from them? I was also being exposed to stray voltage and stray frequencies from the anti-static strap which is extensively documented in the diary industry for making farmers, their families, and their animals sick.

The first person that I knew who committed suicide was in this group. I will always be curious to know if it was caused in part from the toxic exposures that he received during his time in it. He was in the group for many years, as opposed to the three years that I worked there.

In 1999 I went to live in La Palma in the Canary Islands and started to work at an altitude of approximately 7,755 feet. I was working with telescope drive systems that were controlled by industrial computer systems. There are no doubts that sunlight in the right dose is an excellent medication! Living in the Canary Islands did wonders for improving my health. However it was short lived.

I noticed that the longer I was in the position in the Canary Islands, the sicker I was getting. Like many people in this situation, I did not understand what was happening. Today, I do believe that I was actually sitting in the fields of the neighbors cathode ray tube (CRT) television when I was at home. The problem with CRT televisions is that they have extensive fields around them and those fields will pass straight through

walls! Their television was on the other side of the wall from my sofa.

I had also been issued with a laptop computer at work and I was constantly working on it. Email had become a popular form of communication. There were no warnings given about laptop computers and human health. I now know that many laptop computers have unnatural magnetic fields around them, emit electromagnetic interference, and that their displays can induce health problems into the human.

I purchased my first cellphone in La Palma. I had noticed after having it for a while that it would cause strange noises on my stereo system in the car. I now understand this to be the cellphone logging into the cellphone tower every ten minutes or so. The transmission was so powerful from the cellphone that it was interfering with the stereo system!

I lived in two properties in La Palma and the second property was a home that was in the countryside. I only lived in that home for a short period before leaving for my next position in Hawaii. However, I had noticed that my girlfriend was constantly complaining of headaches there and my health was continuing to decline. Today, I suspect that it was the street lights that were outside of the home. Many street lights create a toxic form of light to the human, have stray voltage/currents/frequencies, and they can have strange electromagnetic emissions from them.

I moved to the USA in 2001 and lived in Waimea on the island of Hawaii. I was walking to and from work under the high voltage power lines that ran through the streets there. During that time I had noticed that I was getting very anxious and that if I was placed in a stressful situation that my heartbeat would start to race and my face would flush. I attribute that health effect to the high voltage power lines, as it cleared up when I moved away from Waimea.

Working at 13,796 feet is well known to be harmful to human health and most people on the mountain were in some state of sickness. We were commuting up and down the mountain daily and our bodies were constantly in a state of confusion. I knew from conversations with other staff members that poor health was a feature of daily high altitude commuting. Pilots, air hostesses, and frequent fliers suffer from the same thing.

At 13,796 feet very little grows! It is a barren landscape that is just rocks and cinder. When you work at high altitude you notice that trees stop growing at a very definite altitude. This line of demarcation is called the "Tree Line". It appears to be an effect of radiation exposure. As you increase in altitude, the air gets thinner and less solar radiation filtering is taking place. More energy is in the electromagnetic spectrum and it appears to move outside of what the trees can survive in. You will find very strange growth patterns in the trees near the tree line with unusual branching and weird deformities. For this reason, I advise people to be very careful with high altitude radiation exposure. If there are no trees around at altitude, then you should avoid the sunlight, as it may give you a very strange type of radiation sickness!

In 2003, I joined the astronomy team and moved onto the night shift. I had suspected that living on the mountain for a week and having a week off would be healthier and it was! I also started to build a solar photovoltaic powered home in Hawaii. Everything was going well, until I moved into the home. The home was powered by a modified sine wave inverter system that was ran off a 24 volt battery system that was charged by 8 solar photovoltaic modules. Like most off grid homes, it had "Energy Star" compact florescent lighting (CFL) throughout the home.

I had noticed that there was a constant buzzing on the phone line whenever I would use it. I spoke with the electrician who had installed it and I was advised that it was a feature of off-grid homes. I was developing a wide variety of health issues the longer that I lived in the home. The main health symptom was fatigue. The longer I lived there, the more excessive the fatigue got. I got to the point where I would drink energy drinks and then go to bed and sleep. The drinks were having no effect on me! However, my mating cycle was constantly being triggered.

Today, I realize that the buzzing on the phone line was a combination of dirty electricity on the electrical grounding system combined with radio wave emissions from the electrical wiring. The effect was made worse during the night from the compact florescent lights (CFL) putting harmonics onto the electrical cables and the electromagnetic fields that they emit. I didn't know it at the time, but I had developed electromagnetic hypersensitivity (EHS)!

I knew two other people who lived in off grid solar power homes very well. One was extremely passive aggressive with everyone. His personality was lacking empathy. The other was showing severe symptoms of forgetfulness. When you explore the field of dirty electricity, you find that the off grid homes generally have the poorest power quality. The quality of electricity will vary with the loads on the system. It is likely that this dirty electricity was a source of their problems.

I later installed a wind turbine to supplement the power generated by the solar modules. The wind turbine hardly made any electricity, however, it did make a lot of noise! It would point to the ocean and start up a few hours after sunrise and run until sunset. It would then point to the mountain and start up at midnight and run until dawn. Needless to say, it wreaked havoc with my sleep cycles and this coincided with the worst of the health conditions that showed up in this home. I was not aware of "Wind Turbine Syndrome" and infra-sound health effects at that point.

I developed intestinal pains during working on the night shift and about every two weeks I would get painful cramps that would lead to diarrhea. I did not know it at the time, but it is classical symptoms of shifting solar radiation exposure. It would generally occur on my first day off in sunlight after working a week of nights.

The second person that I knew who committed suicide had worked at this facility. He was a welder. Welders get exposed to significant levels of radio frequencies, stray voltage/currents/frequencies, ultraviolet light and various electromagnetic radiation emissions from their arc welding equipment. Both of the people I have worked with who committed suicide were nice people. Unfortunately, it is well known that electromagnetic radiation exposures can make nice people do strange things that are out of character for them.

In 2006 I changed jobs and went to work in Tucson, Arizona. This signified a move back onto normal utility electricity. The strange thing was, I had noticed the same effect occurring that I had noticed when I started working in the hospital. I was constantly fatigued in this position to the point of almost falling asleep every day in the first few months.

I was spending four hours per day in transportation systems and eight hours at the observatory. The interesting thing is, I had measured the voltage waveform on the electrical system there and it was highly distorted. This distortion creates large amounts of harmonic energy on the electrical system and puts very large fields on the wiring and equipment. I did not realize the implications of that at the time, because I had never been taught that electromagnetic radiation emissions and electrical system harmonics were harmful!

I remember when I saw it that I was surprised. Out at the telescope it was a highly distorted voltage sine wave. However, at the uninterruptible power supply (UPS), it was an almost perfect voltage sine wave. The sine wave got better the closer to the UPS system and worse the further away from it. I suspect that electronically generated sine waves do not travel well over distances, particularly when they are feeding into electronic products. It is likely that the different frequencies of energy in electronically generated AC voltage sine waves start to interact with cables and the electronic products that they supply and this may distort them.

I later hired a contractor to assist with work at the observatory and it was not long before I was hearing the same story from him, he was getting really fatigued too! I attribute the fatigue problems to the electromagnetic fields that were created by the harmonic energy on the electrical system.

At home, my relationship was problematic and within a year we had broken up. All I wanted to do was lay in bed, as my energy levels were so low. I could not sleep much, as I had insomnia constantly. I was getting intestinal pains and diarrhea a few times every month. I had to stop exercising as I would get chest pains and breathing difficulties!

By September 2007 I had developed very strange facial and head pains. They would come and go and I had no idea what it was. I started to go to the doctor and was sent for many tests. No one could tell me what it was. During researching the book "Toxic Electricity", I realized that my seat at the office was next door to the telescope electrical room that contained all of the control systems, WiFi router, networks, and computers! I was sitting next to a laser printer and nearby was the cordless phone. I had been sitting in very large electromagnetic fields every day. The fact that my company wireless laptop computer also had large electromagnetic emissions coming out of it did not help.

The longer that I was in the position, the more aches and pains I was getting. My skin was getting to be so hot and painful that I was having daily baths to try and calm it down. The funny thing was, I looked perfectly normal on the outside! No one would have been aware that my health was failing. Insomnia was a big issue and it was rare that I would get a good nights sleep.

Anxiety became a significant problem and it was getting worse with time. I knew I was being poisoned, I just could not figure out the source of the poison!

I later reported that I had identified a number of environmental health issues to the management team of this facility in 2012, after I had published the book "Toxic Electricity". I did not tell them what I had identified, as I was interested to see if they would want to know. Unfortunately, their response to the problems was silence. Responding with silence to inconvenient truths is a common problem in the workplace today and is a major problem with the prevalence of sick building syndrome (SBS). Many managers know that their facilities are causing their staff to be sick, but simply stay silent about it. What I found most concerning about this is that it was an Ivy League college and university that specializes in human health!

I joined the solar industry in 2008 and by this time fatigue, insomnia, occasional intestinal pains and diarrhea, hot skin, and general aches and pains throughout my body had become something that I had accepted as aging. My doctor was informing me that it was a normal aspect of aging, everyone is the same! Staying awake on the job was getting to be a significant problem.

I eventually started to see the doctor for medication to keep me awake in order to keep working. I was taking a medication called "Provigil". It keeps you awake for exactly sixteen hours from the point of taking it. The military issue it to the troops during wars to prevent the troops from sleeping when they are under attack. It is an amazing medication and worked well for me. However, it does not make the original problems go away, it simply masks them. It also costs approximately $400 per month!

Needless to say, I was not looking for a tablet, I was looking for a cure!

I had started to develop blotchy patches of skin on my buttocks. They were not painful or sore. I had noticed them in the mirror after showering one day. They were there for months. I saw the doctor about them and they did not know what would cause it. Today, I suspect that it was the company cellphone electromagnetic emissions that were causing them, as I would keep the mobile phone in my back pocket. They cleared up after I left that company and I have never seen them since. The blotchy skin effect is reported by people who have Electromagnetic Hypersensitivity.

During the development of the book "Toxic Electricity", I analyzed the environment that I was working in. I was working in a cubicle desk that was surrounded by other workers who had cellphones and wireless computer systems. My desk was very close to the electrical room that housed all of the computer network equipment for the building and the wireless router. The high voltage overhead utility power lines and poles in the street were approximately 30 feet from my desk! The airport was across the road and there would have been extensive RADAR and radio wave emissions from it. There may have been infra-sound and pollution issues as well. The company used radio frequency identification (RFID) controlled doors and I would pass through these perhaps 100 times per day to get between departments. I was also sitting near to the transmitting RFID door sensor.

In 2009 I commissioned a very large utility solar power system over two months. It was an interesting experience that was setting the stage for finding the cure that I was looking for.

During the two months of commissioning, I had noticed some very strange behaviors in the people involved with the project. I was seeing aggressiveness, fatigue, confusion and forgetfulness. I was also seeing habitual lying over commissioning issues that were showing up and that appeared to be caused by pressure for the project to be perceived as successful by the company management team. In conversations with the staff, they were telling me that they were not sleeping well and that they were having aches and pains throughout their bodies. Very similar conditions to my own!

One day, after spending the entire day working around the high voltage transformers, electronic power inverter systems and solar modules, I noticed that my smell was off. At the time, I was in the 24,000 volt switching center at the site and I could smell smoke when there was no smoke. The most amount of electrical power was in here, as it feeds into the electrical utility transmission system. It was a sunny day with millions of watts of electronically generated harmonic electricity flowing through the room.

I was absolutely convinced that something was on fire and the people that I was with were telling me that they could not smell it. I also appeared to be intoxicated. Later that day, I found that I could not stop drinking due to an insatiable thirst! I had been drinking during the day and I did not appear to be dehydrated, my urine was not dark nor was I sunburned as I had sunscreen on, sunglasses, a wide brimmed hard hat, and a whole body arc flash suit. Everything appeared to be back to normal the next day.

During research for my books, I found that these symptoms are listed as radio wave sickness (RWS). I was not surprised, as the power plant was producing excessive harmonics and nobody had warned me about the dangers of high powered electronic utility equipment that has excessive harmonic energy on it.

After leaving this project, I soon discovered that I could not remember computer passwords, phone numbers, alarm codes, and basic mathematics was difficult for me. It was clear that I had received a toxic brain exposure from the high powered electronic utility equipment. Nikola Tesla documents having a similar experience during his research and development.

I started to develop books on solar power systems and that led to the discovery of the "multiple-Sun" effect. The multiple-Sun effect occurs anywhere that there are solar reflections taking place. Solar power systems with their reflective glass surfaces create it. I knew the effect was important and I started to develop it further. I found that it also occurs in city environments where there are large amounts of glass in buildings. It is particularly bad around glass covered tower buildings.

The multiple-Sun effect significantly raises the radiation levels in the human environment to above the radiation levels of Space. Bingo! I had discovered that I had developed radiation sickness over the years of extended exposure to radiation sources.

I also stopped taking the medications. I had been taking Provigil for the daytime and over the counter sleeping tablets to counteract the insomnia symptoms. This over the counter sleep medication was a range of melatonin, diphenhydramine, and doxylamine succinate. The doctor has prescribed Seroquel, but I found that it made me feel really bad for the first hour in the morning.

The interesting thing is, it is commonly reported in the USA that approximately 50% of the population is taking prescription medications! I had noticed on my travels that many people that I have worked with are routinely taking medications. I was not alone in this lifestyle that had developed over the years. Unfortunately, many USA children are also in the same situation.

Within days I went into really severe drugs withdrawal. I literally could not get out of bed for a few days as I felt so bad. Flu like symptoms followed by really bad headaches for about two weeks that would not respond to medication. I had never experienced this before!

It slowly cleared up which led me to the understanding that if you take medications long term, then your mind and body will go toxic. The interesting thing was, my thought patterns changed! A calm mind replaced a mind that was constantly active with various thoughts. My insomnia also slowly cleared up. As such, it is better to avoid the medications if you can.

After doing the work with the development of the multiple-Sun effect in 2010, I knew that it was wise to balance it out and to spend a corresponding amount of time out of the Sun. For six months, I avoided sunlight. A few weeks into this process, I got extremely ill with flu like symptoms. My heart beat was fluctuating and I had intense pains throughout my body. It was so bad that I thought that I was going to die! It lasted a few days and then slowly got better. It was clear at this point that I was in radiation withdrawal. About a month into the withdrawal I had my blood tested and everything was showing normal levels.

Extreme fatigue followed for a few months and that eventually cleared up. I noticed that several weeks into the withdrawal process that my body was reacting to sunlight exposure, if I spent time outside in the Sun, then I would have a big headache the next day.

I went to view Niagara falls with my friends and we rode right up to the bright white wall of water on the Maid of the Mist. For me, it was like drinking several beers, it made me develop symptoms of intoxication!

As time went by, my pains started to subside. Eventually, they disappeared! Today, after years of random aches and pains, I am pain free.

After several months of avoiding the Sun, I had my blood tested again and it had gone low in both vitamin B12 and vitamin D. My diet had not changed, the only thing that had changed was my sunlight exposure. The vitamin D deficiency was expected, as it is well documented as being a photosynthesis vitamin. There was plenty of meat and fish in my diet for sources of B12, so being low on B12 was a surprise. So I concluded that the B12 deficiency was related to the lack of Sun exposure.

It is interesting to note that in Autistic children, vitamin B12 injections have been shown to significantly reduce their symptoms. I do currently believe that both Autism and Attention Deficit Disorder (ADD) are electromagnetic diseases.

I started to get 15 minutes of Sun per day, which is the current guidelines for maintaining adequate vitamin D levels. Much to my surprise, I eventually got to a period where extreme fatigue showed up and all that I wanted to do was sleep every day. My vitamin D and B12 levels appeared to continue to decline and had brought on the symptoms of Seasonal Affect Disorder (SAD). I increased the sunlight exposure time to an hour per day in the shade and that eventually fixed it.

Just for curiosity, I actually started to sunbathe and found that at two hours per day, the aches and pains came back. They were simply fixed by staying out of the Sun for a few days. I eventually established that my outdoor solar radiation levels are at 1 hour per day in the shade in sunny Arizona to maintain good health. My genetics are a mix of Irish and English with relatively white skin. My skin today is a golden brown. If you have darker skin, then your daily requirements for solar radiation exposure will be higher due to the pigmentation. I later realized that the aches and pains may have been caused by the high wireless radiation levels outside, as my plants were showing deformities in that area. Some parts of my garden have wireless radiation levels of approximately 700 millivolts per meter, which is considered very high by most electromagnetic radiation researchers. In the National Park forest, the wireless energy meter reads zero.

At this point, the main problem that I was showing was occasional fatigue. It was the kind of fatigue that makes you want to take a nap in the middle of the day. During research for the book "Toxic Electricity" I had realized that people who report electromagnetic hypersensitivity generally report fatigue. I started to research my human body voltage and found that there was a large AC waveform riding on my body. Turning off my home electrical circuits eliminated it. I also discovered that my tiled flooring in the home was electrified with stray voltage/current/frequency from the electrical utility neutral and started to wear slippers when home to prevent coming into contact with it. I changed all of my light bulbs from compact florescent lights (CFL) to conventional filament lights. I tested the CFL's and found that they had unnatural spectrums of light and radio wave emissions. I switched over to a diet rich in organic fresh fruit and vegetables and turned off the cell phone. These actions brought up my energy levels.

I should mention that due to my knowledge of how utility power companies willfully mislead the public, during the Fukushima nuclear disaster I changed my diet over to dried and canned food in March 2011 to avoid the surge of radiation contaminated food in the USA food system. During the following nine months, I noticed that my skin started to develop problems on my elbows with rough, dry, and brittle skin. My teeth started to decay, and I was getting indigestion and stomach problems. Heart burn and acid reflux was an issue and I was constantly taking antacids to alleviate the symptoms. These problems fixed themselves after a few months of eating fresh organic food.

I concluded that extended exposure to preserved food is harmful to human health and the health problems can be simply fixed by eating fresh organic food.

I had noticed that the occasional fatigue completely cleared up when I went camping in National Parks, which I would do at least once per year. To clear the occasional fatigue up, I suspected that I was going to have to move to a different area, due to the high radiation levels around my property from the three cell phone towers that are approximately between 2,000 feet to 2,300 feet from my home. I had planted trees and plants around my property when I purchased it and I knew that they would eventually reduce the radiation levels by absorbing it.

Watching the plants grow over the years led me to the understanding that things were not growing correctly in the garden. The extensive indoor plant experiments that I was performing showed me that the electromagnetic radiation environment of the entire home was extremely unnatural, as even my control plants were deforming! I had many

Dieffenbachia (Dumb Cane) plants in the home and every one was deformed! There were zones around the outside of the home that were showing stress and growth problems in the plants. These were the entire west side of the home and the entire north east side of the home where the utility gas and electrical equipment was located. The northwest part of the garden was the worst and there were areas that I had noticed that the plants would die when placed there. It did not matter what type of plant I planted in these locations, they would die after several months.

I took all of my wireless devices out of service in summertime 2012 and had the utility company change out the automatic meter reader (AMR) for a conventional mechanical electric meter on both my home and the neighbors home. This appears to have cured some of the growth problems that I was seeing in my plants. It was clear that the utility company and my wireless devices had inadvertently turned my home and garden area into the equivalent of an antenna park! It improved the occasional fatigue, but did not fully clear it up. I did get very sore and sensitive teeth in the weeks following removing the wireless products, as did my neighbors. It appeared to be a withdrawal symptom from the wireless radiation. In summertime 2013 I had the first ever fruits that the garden had produced from a peach and a pomegranate tree. It was obvious that the wireless radiation exposures had been causing these trees to abort their fruit development in the previous years.

Many people report problems with metal coil mattresses. I checked mine out and found that it was acting as an antenna system for AC electricity and radio waves! I changed out my metal coil mattress to a latex mattress to see if that would help. It improved my sleep, but did not appear to improve the occasional fatigue.

I tried the "Earthing" health technique for two reasons. I wanted to assess it for the book "Toxic Electricity" and I thought that it may clear up the fatigue. I saw my back tingle for about a week in the area where I was in contact with the earthing cable, so it definitely was doing something. However, as time went on I got the most severe bad back that I have ever had. It was in the base of my spine and badly affected my walking! It took a few weeks to clear up. Then I went into the worst period of heart arrhythmia that I have ever experienced! Fearing a heart attack, I decided to stop the technique. I tested the cable and found that it was acting as an antenna system and had a wide range of frequencies on it! The technique did not work for me, but there are people who say that it does work.

People had commented over the years that when they would enter my home that there was a strange odor. I had wondered for a long time where this odor was coming from, as I had noticed it myself from time to time. It was apparent when coming into the home after it had been locked up for several hours. I found that my kitchen island had an in-line sewer vent valve installed into it. These valves allow air to enter into the sewer system from the home and prevent the sewer gas from escaping. When the in-line vent valve ages, it may start to leak sewer gas. Replacing this fixed the odor problem. If you have one of these valves in your home, you should pay attention to it as sewer gas is explosive and poisonous!

I followed Dr. John Nash Ott's advice and installed ultraviolet (UV) transmitting plastic in the areas of my home where I spend my daytime. When compared to the crystal clear UV transmitting acrylic windows, my double glazed glass windows look green and dim! This heavily filtered colored light from the low-E double glazed glass windows appears to have been contributing to the fatigue issues that I was seeing. Using "full spectrum" glazing appears to have significantly reduced the occasional fatigue problem.

The health benefits that I observed during the initial few weeks of testing ultraviolet transmitting acrylic windows were:

- **Excellent daytime energy levels.**
- **Wonderful sleep cycle.**
- **Improved mental functioning.**
- **Brighter indoor environment.**
- **Indoor colors are vivid.**
- **The computer is more pleasant to work with. It appears to have significantly reduced the dry eyes and chapped lips that it gave me with long periods of use.**
- **Fruits ripen faster in the full spectrum light.**
- **Good health.**

In the first month that I installed this I did see some interesting aches and pains. My left ankle and my right elbow were aching for no reason whatsoever. I then got some intestinal pains that I have not had before. They cleared up after a few weeks and appeared to be due to the changes that were taking place in my body.

After the initial surge in health, I started getting the desire to occasionally nap again at lunchtime. I have established that I get full health whenever I go camping in National Parks or travel to areas that are rural with very low cell phone reception. While I have always associated good health with low cell phone reception, I do spend more time outside around nature on these trips.

I increased my outdoor time to two hours around solar noon in the shade. Generally I will read a book during this time. I will get a little direct sunlight exposure also, typically half an hour. This really brought up my energy levels.

This leads me to conclude that exposure to the peak in solar radiation that occurs around solar noon is essential to good health. My daily solar radiation exposure is to sit near to my shady ultraviolet transmitting full spectrum acrylic window while I develop my research and then to go out around solar noon for a couple of hours in the shade reading. I'll take a stroll around the garden in the direct sunlight during that time.

I moved my computer next to the shady ultraviolet transmitting window. When I work on it during the daytime, I now have the outdoors in my field of view. This enables my eyes, face and hands to get full spectrum daylight exposure all day long. My daytime light environment is now in tune with thousands of

years of evolution. One could say that I have finally achieved resonance with the daylight environment!

I also discovered that the gas company installed an automatic meter reader (AMR) radiation transmitting device at my property during this time. I do not know exactly when it was installed, but I asked around and it appears that it was installed sometime in January 2013. It was the reason why my health took a step back. The gas company installed them throughout the community, as I could see the same shiny AMR meters at other properties in the neighborhood. I tested it and it was emitting a radiation pulse every several seconds. The previous gas meter had no detectable radiation pulses coming from it. I am now watching my plants in that area to see if they are going to deform, go dormant or die.

To reduce the toxic effects of this, I have now moved my desk as far away from the AMR gas meters that I can in the home. It is simply the prudent thing to do. The World Health Organization class wireless transmitting devices as "Possibly Carcinogenic". There are no shortage of people who have traced their health problems to these devices and one can only wonder why they have not been banned. Moving further away from the AMR transmitters increased my energy levels which tells me that they are affecting my health. The symptoms that I have observed are:

- January: Fatigue.
- February: Fatigue, waking up feeling hung over and lethargic.

- March: Fatigue, waking up feeling hung over and lethargic, fuzzy thinking and concentration problems.

- April: I abandoned my bed and started to sleep on the floor. I also increased the electromagnetic screening around the transmitting AMR meters. This reduced the severity of the symptoms.

I notified both the gas company and the Federal Communication Commission (FCC) that they were causing harmful biological interference at my property and to remove the AMR transmitting devices from the vicinity of my home.

In March 2013 I started to get really sick with classic radio wave sickness symptoms. This is how the sickness progressed:

- Day 1 - Fuzzy thinking.
- Day 2 - Dizziness, fuzzy thinking, headaches.
- Day 3 - Dizziness, fuzzy thinking, headaches, insomnia.
- Day 4 & 5 - Dizziness, fuzzy thinking, headaches, insomnia, fatigue.

I had seen this range of symptoms appear with a similar rapid progression back in summertime 2012 when I went to stay in a mountaintop forest vacation area. When I researched the location from satellites I found that I had been staying just a few hundred meters from a large antenna park that had cell phone towers and multiple radome installations in it! The interesting thing was, my girlfriend showed a different rate of progression. She was symptom free until the fourth day when she started showing headaches, insomnia and fatigue. We were both relieved to leave that location and our symptoms rapidly subsided within hours of departing the area.

It was clearly radio wave sickness that had shown up, but what was causing it? My best guess was that I had moved into a hotspot of radiation and that it was affecting me. It was the correct assumption. I had been given a printer to repair and was using it daily to test it. I had noticed that it had built in WiFi but was not using it. I tested the printer with my radio frequency meter and there was a large field of wireless radiation around it! I had been sitting just 2 feet away from the printer in a 1,000 mV/m radiation field daily and this was consistent with the symptoms that had shown up. It appears that wireless network printers exhibit a similar behavior to wireless network routers and continually fill the area with microwave radiation. It is for this reason that you should not sit near to devices like this. The best way is simply not to have wireless devices of any kind.

I had noticed that the acrylic windows were reacting to infra-sound. A pulse of energy would hit them and make them vibrate. It is very noticeable at my home and lasts less than a second. There is no wind present when I have seen this occur. Out in the desert is a military bombing range that generates sonic booms. When I worked on Kitt Peak, I would hear the sonic booms frequently and they would shake the buildings. It appears that I am now detecting them at my home with my acrylic windows! This is concerning, as infra-sound is well known for its ability to make people sick and sonic booms are known to cause heart problems.

In May 2013 I found that my toilets were electrified with stray voltage/current/frequency. When I would urinate into them this would make the drain wet and electrify them from the stray voltage/current/frequency in the street! I was curious and tested my showers and found that when the drain gets wet, it electrifies the shower! This is a concerning development, as it means that there are many toilets and drains out there that are electrified. This is consistent with some trips that I took to the doctors several years ago with urethra problems that the doctor could not diagnose. I suspect that the stray voltage/current/frequency issue was much higher during that period. I only saw it for one year and then it spontaneously cleared up. Needless to say, now I know that my drains are electrified, I no longer urinate into my toilets. This action increased my energy levels. I did see quite severe headaches occur during the following two weeks that gradually subsided.

High activity muscle building exercise was a step that I had wanted to introduce for quite some time. I was reluctant to start doing it while I was dealing with and characterizing the earlier issues. I have always walked for exercise during this recovery process but I wanted to introduce a daily exercise regimen that made me really sweaty! Walking is not really exercise, as it does not work the entire body. This was evidenced by my weight increasing from 154 pounds in 2009 to 192 pounds in 2013. During that period I had led a sedentary life with most of my time spent at home. I started to follow a DVD workout routine every day. I lost 6 pounds in the first ten days! The thing that was very noticeable was that my hunger subsided and that I was content with smaller portions. My body shape change was evident as was my increase in muscle mass. After twenty days my weight had stabilized at 184 pounds and it was obvious that my fat was in the process of being converted into muscle, as the exercise routine had become enjoyable and my strength had significantly increased. By thirty days my stamina had developed and I was able to fully perform each exercise routine. After sixty days I had muscle definition in my arms and legs and the majority of my fat had converted to muscle with a weight of 182 pounds. It is clear that it does take approximately 90 days of daily strength exercise to take the human from an atrophied state to a lean and muscular body.

While I was setting up a structured water plant experiment, it caused me to investigate what exactly was in my drinking water filter. I had been advised by numerous people in Tucson to filter my water, as they believed that the drinking water was contaminated by industrial and mining activities in the area. I thought that I was carbon filtering my water. However, when I checked the water filter box, I found that there were ion exchange resin beads in addition to carbon. It appears that since 2007 that I was drinking carbon filtered ion exchanged water! I checked the filters out on the internet and sure enough, I found many complaints about them from people who had been made ill by using them. Naturally, I switched my drinking water back to standard faucet water from the utility company. Over the following weeks I saw my energy levels increase.

The gas company did eventually remove the biologically harmful AMR meter from my home. However, they refused to remove the one on the neighbors home just 15 feet away! I had actually requested that they remove four of their transmitting meters from within 100 feet of my bedrooms, but only the one on my home was changed for a non-transmitting meter. The gas company knows that these transmitting meters make me sick, but are okay with that state of affairs. It is clearly a case of willful biological assault with known biologically harmful radio frequency devices that the military weaponized as they were so good at making the enemy sick! And it is happening at my home which represents my greatest financial investment! My home is not a place of safe refuge and this is a violation of the USA Declaration of Independence.

Today I have health that I thought impossible to achieve just a few months ago in this home. While I have been able to alleviate some of the symptoms that showed up when the AMR transmitting gas meter was installed throughout my community, the symptom of occasional daytime fatigue is proving difficult to shake off and is in line with living in an unnaturally high radio frequency field. The biological toxins that I am being exposed to concern me. It is well known in the electromagnetic community that people who are showing mild symptoms of electromagnetic stress typically have blood composition that matches the people who are showing severe stress. The blood composition tends to be abnormal either way!

Heart arrhythmia and insomnia eventually showed up when I was sleeping on the floor. It was likely a combination of extended exposure to the transmitting utility meters in the area and the summertime stray voltage levels increasing on the concrete floor that I was sleeping on. This required a change in direction to seek good health.

I moved back onto the master bed and I am now experimenting with applying an indirect DC voltage field to the human during sleep and a direct DC voltage exposure during daytime activities. The heart arrhythmia and insomnia has subsided and this technique is showing promising health results with alleviating the final health symptom of occasional fatigue. It is clear from the many plant growth experiments that I have performed with the Dieffenbachia plant that an atmospheric DC voltage has gone missing in the modern world and this lack of DC atmospheric voltage is having far reaching consequences for all life where it is not present. It appears that a great biological price has been paid by the modern masses for the convenience of tall man-made structures, electricity and wireless radiation.

Ultimately, it appears that I have now reached the point where I have to move home. There are simply too many environmental problems that I cannot rectify at my home. My impression from dealing with the utilities and government regulators is that my home is simply typical of the average American home! I find this very concerning. There comes a point where you have to acknowledge that some environmental variables are outside of your control and you have to move to rectify them. These are:

- Utility company AMR radiation transmitting meter emissions. (Gas utility, Arizona Corporation Commission and the Federal Communications Commission refuses to remove them from within 100 feet of my bedrooms).

- Stray voltage/current/frequency on my tiled flooring, toilets, baths and showers from the electrical utility system in the street. (Electrical utility and Arizona Corporation Commission refuses to fix it).

- Neighbors wireless radiation emissions including their transmitting utility meters. (Gas utility, Arizona Corporation Commission and the Federal Communications Commission refuses to remove the neighbor's AMR gas meter that is just 15 feet from my home)

- Sonic boom infra-sound waves. (The military bombing range is not moving any time soon).

- Missing DC atmospheric voltage gradient. (It appears to be an effect of tall man-made structures, atmospheric wireless radiation overloading and the utility systems in the area.)

The utilities and corporate governments are fully aware that they are making many people in their own populations sick. They are completely okay with this. Your sickness is nothing more than an "Inconvenient Truth" to their profit making empires that they have created. The causes of human sickness will be willfully ignored while massive profits are abundant. This is evidenced by the utilities not removing their toxic pulsing wireless transmitting devices from homes that have sick people in them who are unsuccessfully trying to get them removed. It is simply a blatant violation of the basic human right to a healthy and safe life.

So how is my health today in 2013? I have definitely seen the effects that Dr. John Nash Ott talked about in his books and I have also seen them in people that I have worked with. I have had large exposures to these electromagnetic field effects for 27 years now and I am relatively healthy. I managed to recover the majority of my memory, but I do not think it will ever fully recover back to what it was prior to 2009. The exposures that I got from the high powered utility electronic generation system were extremely biologically toxic to the human mind. I do not take any medications nor vitamin supplements and I eat mostly organic food and drink utility faucet water. I keep track of my daily outdoor sunlight exposure to make sure that I get sufficient daily exposure in the shade in a natural green environment. I now spend every day in rooms that have shady "Full Spectrum" acrylic windows. I keep my nighttime lighting low and use 120 volt soft white filament light bulbs in my home.

In 2009 the doctors could not diagnose what was wrong with me, they were telling me that I was getting old and it was a normal aspect of aging. I now know that they were misleading me, as what I had was not a normal aspect of aging. My health was at its worst in 2009 and I could only work due to taking prescription drugs. Without the drugs I would have been constantly in bed with fatigue day and night and unable to work. I no longer need any drugs nor supplements of any kind and I have excellent sleep patterns. My health is 90% recovered and I can fully recover it by going into rural areas that have little pollution. I do have to conclude at this point that the reason why I cannot get 100% health at my home is due to incorrect human environmental conditions.

This matches the growth patterns that I observe in the Dieffenbachia (Dumb Cane) plants. After two years of growing these at my home, I can only get them to grow normally by connecting them to a 1.5 volt DC battery! The rest of my Dieffenbachia plants are all showing strange growth patterns.

Based on what I see with these plants, I have to conclude that modern cities and suburban areas have a level of biological toxicity associated with them. This toxicity is increasing with each year of the wireless revolution. This matches what we are seeing in the children. Autism is an accelerating disease in the children and there are no doubts today that electromagnetic interference exposures are driving it. The children are like the "coalminers canaries", when they are not developing properly, you know you have got some really serious human environmental problems!

I think that 90% of full health is the best that a person can obtain in a suburban environment. I think that it may be even lower in a city environment due to the wireless radiation overloading and the tall structures, and "Full City Health" may only be at 80%. The only way a person can obtain 100% health in a wireless radiation society is to go to rural areas. I do believe that I have obtained at this point what I call "Full Suburban Health". I do prefer what I call "Full Rural Health" and my future plans revolve around moving to a rural area that has little wireless radiation pollution and no tall structures. Unfortunately, such areas are rapidly disappearing and there is no escaping satellite transmissions.

I do consider Tucson, Arizona to be a biologically toxic town as many properties have three AMR radiation transmitting utility meters on them. Add in the sonic boom infra-sound emissions, the missing DC atmospheric voltage and the stray voltage problems from the dry desert electrical grounding systems and it is a really toxic mess!

If you are considering moving to Tucson, I would recommend that you go to a different town that does not have these biological problems. Tucson has a high rate of Autism that is likely related to these problems.

National Parks offer the ability to assess if your health symptoms are being caused by electrical exposures, transmitter systems, tall structures and window glazing in your environment. Most transmitter systems are banned from National Parks and that includes cell phone towers. So take a camping trip in a remote part of the National Park and engage in outdoor activities for a few weeks and see if your health improves there. Be careful though, as you may initially go into withdrawal! The withdrawal will be similar to cold and flu symptoms and should clear up after a week or so.

There is only one reason why I am relatively healthy today and that is because I detoxed from the radiation exposures after discovering that I had radiation sickness.

So, as you can see, I have had quite a journey through the realms of human health issues. My conclusion is that the majority of ailments that humans suffer from are caused by incorrect environmental exposures. Both sunlight and electrical systems are sources of radiation exposures and you need to be aware of your exposure to these.

You should spend time characterizing your body and establish the correct daily level of outdoor sunlight exposure for it. You should also characterize your electrical environment and reduce your exposures as much as possible to electrical systems and products. You should only have the exposures that are absolutely necessary in order to do what you need to do. The more exposures you have to electricity then the more likely it is to impact your health. These health effects appear in most people as general poor health and compromised mental functioning.

Regarding children, you should avoid purchasing electrical, electronic and wireless toys for them. It is preferable to also turn off the electrical circuit in their bedroom. Developing children should not be sleeping in rooms that have electricity in them. Do not purchase a television or laptop computer for their rooms, as the electromagnetic fields are too large for their developing cells to cope with in the long term. With developing children you should be keeping their environment as natural as possible.

It is preferable to arrange your rooms and use common sense so that you are not exposed to easily avoidable electromagnetic fields. Some simple steps are:

- Do not walk barefoot on conductive flooring that has stray voltage/current/frequency on it.

- Do not urinate into toilets that have stray voltage/current/frequency on the water.

- Keep chairs away from walls.

- Avoid putting chairs within 10 feet of a television in all directions.

- Be aware of what products are on the other side of the walls.

- Do not put chairs near to large appliances like cookers, microwave ovens, refrigerators, washers and dryers.

- Stay away from electrical fuse boards and utility meters.

- Be aware of what is under the floor on upper story's and avoid the electromagnetic hotspots that may appear in the floor.

- Use wooden furniture.

- Sleep on a natural foam mattress.

- Your bedroom should be free of electricity and electrical, electronic and wireless products.

- Do not use radioactive americium ionizing smoke detectors, have optical ones instead.

- Do not use wireless products.

- Use only the electrical and electronic products that you need. Unplug them when not in use.

- Use filament light bulbs.

- Be aware of the transmitters in your local neighborhood.

- Pay attention to the locations of streetlights and power poles near your home.

Good health for most people is easy to achieve and it just takes some simple adjustments in lifestyle. The adjustments are far easier than expensive visits to the doctor and mentally challenged children.

"The only people mad at you for speaking the TRUTH are those living a lie. Keep speaking it."

Unknown

<u>Summary</u>

I find it unfortunate that I have worked with a number of professional electrical engineers in the USA that I can only describe their conduct as extremely unprofessional and blatantly illegal. Working with them alerted me to wonder what exactly it was that they were trying to hide.

When you see a large number of utility workers disregarding the laws of the USA and demonstrating a willful lack of caring for the health and safety of the people that they are responsible for, you do start to wonder why they do this? The development of this book revealed what they were up to.

The adoption of electricity led to the regular unnatural exposure of electromagnetic interference in the human mind and body. This corresponded to an increase in illness, disease, cancer, and mental health issues. New illnesses and diseases were born with the progression of electricity.

The reason why I was able to write this book is because I have inadvertently taken the human mind and body through almost the entire range of electromagnetic exposures that are possible without dying or becoming diseased. There are no doubts that dirty electricity has toxic effects on both the human mind and body. The most toxic exposures that I have had are from transmitter systems, stray voltage/current/frequency and electromagnetic fields.

This is consistent with health problems that were documented in Nikola Tesla. Nikola Tesla had many health problems during his life and he appeared to die of dementia. He had occurrences of amnesia and numerous mental breakdowns during his life. He was known for his phobias and his love of pigeons. However, no love interest was ever documented in his life. The book "Tesla: Man Out of Time" by Margaret Cheney extensively discusses his health problems and is an interesting read.

Sick kids? You should take a good look at their electromagnetic environment. It is likely that it is having a significant affect on their health. Children who are inadvertently sitting in fields of unnatural electromagnetic interference may not develop correctly. The same is true for children who do not get the correct daily outdoor exposure to sunlight in a green environment.

Insomnia? Take a look at your lighting products. Avoid the energy star lighting products and use filament light bulbs instead. Keep nighttime lighting low and just sufficient for the application. Reduce your television and computer time. Make sure that you are not inadvertently sitting in electromagnetic fields. Wireless transmitter systems can cause insomnia and you should turn them off.

Fatigue? Your home and office wiring may be radiating radio waves, magnetic fields, and electric fields into your environment. Simply switch off your electrical circuits to reduce your exposure to these. Avoid living and working near to transmitter systems and go back to wired products instead of cordless. Wear slippers inside your home to prevent contact with electrically conductive flooring. Wear insulated shoes when outside of the home to prevent contact with stray voltage/current/frequency.

Random aches and pains? You may need to hibernate for 40 days and nights to detoxify from the radiation sources that you have been exposed to over the years. Avoid sitting near to electrical cables and limit your time on laptop computers and cellphones. Avoid sitting next to windows that have a direct view of the Sun.

Low vitamin D and B12? You will need to increase your daily outdoor sunlight exposure in a green natural environment. Remember not to wear glasses nor sunglasses, no contact lenses, no sunscreen, no lipstick and no make-up. It is a good idea to go for a daily walk in a park or the countryside in order to obtain this exposure.

Sexual addiction? Certain types of electromagnetic field exposures trigger the human mating cycle. You should turn off your electrical and electronic products and install filament light bulbs to see if it clears up. If it does, you will know that one of your products is triggering it. It may be your electrical system at work, so take a camping vacation in the forest in the National Park and see if it clears up. If it does, you will know that it is environmental. You may be walking or driving past power poles that have high electromagnetic interference emissions, so change your route. It may also be coming from the transportation systems that you use.

Irregular heartbeats? You may be in electromagnetic fields that are interfering with the electrical system of the heart. Reduce your electromagnetic radiation exposure and avoid walking near power lines. Stray voltage/current/frequency exposure and radio frequency fields can cause arrhythmia and you should avoid them. Sonic booms and infra-sound are known to interfere with the heart and you should avoid these exposures.

Mental health issues, relationship problems or anxiety? The human mind is constantly adapting to the environmental conditions that it is placed into. When in an unnatural environment, then the thinking will also be unnatural. Unnatural thoughts and behaviors will take over and they will seem normal to you. Ensure your environmental conditions are correct for clear thinking.

Aggression or headaches? Over exposure to electromagnetic radiation causes this. Simply reduce your exposure to fix it.

Eye problems? Artificial lighting sources can cause this. · Sit facing shady windows with natural views to prevent it. Radio frequency exposures can cause cataracts and you should examine if your environment is inadvertently exposing you to transmitting systems.

Hot skin, facial pains or blotchy skin? Electromagnetic fields cause a reaction in the skin that can make it exhibit a hot sensation and pins and needles pains. Remove yourself from the electromagnetic fields. Cell phones are known to cause the blotchy skin effect where they are kept against the body. Carry your cell phone in a bag away from the body. Man-made ultraviolet light emissions from lighting products are known to cause skin problems and they may be reduced or eliminated by changing to a different lighting product.

Hearing things? You may have electromagnetic hearing that is documented as a high pitched noise or a low frequency hum. Change your electromagnetic environment.

The modern electrical system presents a high risk of toxic exposures to the human. Some electrical systems are relatively clean, while others present the health risks of high levels of electromagnetic interference exposure. Many products have been made that are unintentional radio and microwave transmitters. Some electrical products test fine when new, but may degrade with age into toxic products.

Electrical wiring and products in the home and office should be minimal. You should consider only having it in the areas that need it, such as the kitchen, bathroom and an entertainment room. Limit wiring in other areas to lighting and one socket in each room. Each room should be on its own circuit breaker and the fuse board should have a filter installed into it. The wiring should not be run close to where people are sleeping.

We appear to be witnessing the development of the next generation of nature. It is the electromagnetically hardened version. The humans that survive this era of rapid genetic change across all species will most likely go on to found the future generation of humans.

Unfortunately, we will witness extensive development problems, sickness, disease, and premature death in the humans that are not destined for this future. That is where we are today and it is comparable to ethnic cleansing of the global population. Personally, I find this situation unacceptable because it is clearly avoidable.

I have every expectation that in the future, electricity will be regarded in the same way that asbestos and smoking are viewed today. The electrification of the ground that we walk on can only be described as the actions of an insane race of people. Stray voltage/current/frequency effects, biological field coupling, toxic electric lighting products, willingly electrifying the environment with radio and microwaves, and developing radioactive energy sources will be documented by future historians as the peak of human insanity.

Energy fields define who we are as humans. If you are in environments that are creating positive energy, then you will have excellent mental and physical health. If you are in environments where the energy levels are negative, then you will fall into poor mental and physical health. Unfortunately, modern society has created far more negative energy fields and finding good mental and physical health is becoming increasingly difficult.

The majority of human illness and disease appears to have its root cause in:

- Unnatural radiation exposures.
- Nutritionally deficient foods.

- Drinking mineral deficient water.

- Toxic exposures from medications and supplements.

- Toxic air exposures.

Feng Shui is the study of positive energy in the human environment. It literally means wind and water. The people who developed Feng Shui understood that human emotions and health were governed by their environments. If you are feeling ill or having emotional issues, you should apply the science of Feng Shui to your environment as it will probably help a lot. You cannot go wrong by having an environment that has the science of Feng Shui applied to it.

I feel that John Lennon's quote is appropriate for what I found when I researched this book:

Our society is run by insane people for insane objectives. I think we're being run by maniacs for maniacal ends and I think I'm liable to be put away as insane for expressing that. That's what's insane about it.

John Lennon

One has to wonder if the time has come to implement the Declaration of Independence to put a stop to the fraudulent corporate and government behaviors that are stealing the future from the children?

Life, Liberty and the pursuit of Happiness.--That to secure these rights, Governments are instituted among

Men, deriving their just powers from the consent of the governed, --That whenever any Form of Government becomes destructive of these ends, it is the Right of the People to alter or to abolish it, and to institute new Government, laying its foundation on such principles and organizing its powers in such form, as to them shall seem most likely to effect their Safety and Happiness.

USA Declaration of Independence

For more information on light, I can recommend the book "Toxic Light". Human health is an extensive field and we have only covered one small aspect of it here. As such, I can recommend the book "Toxic Health" to people who want to understand the many aspects that go into being healthy.

I hope that you enjoyed the book and I wish you the very best of health.

"Wisdom and money can get you almost anything, but only wisdom can save your life."

Ecclesiastes 7:12

References

- AARP: http://www.aarp.org/
- Amateur Radio Wiki: http://www.amateur-radio-wiki.net/
- Ansel Adams
- AntennaSearch.com: http://www.antennasearch.com/
- Arizona Daily Star: http://azstarnet.com/
- BBC News: http://www.bbc.co.uk/news/
- Berenson-Allen Center for Noninvasive Brain Stimulation: http://tmslab.org/
- Breastcancer.org: http://www.breastcancer.org/
- Camilla Rees, MBA
- "Challenging the Chip: Labor Rights and Environmental Justice in the Global Electronics Industry." book by Ted Smith, David A. Sonnenfeld, David Naguib Pellow, and Jim Hightower.
- "Color and Light: Their Effects on Plants, Animals and People." book by Dr. John Nash Ott
- "Cross Currents: The Perils of Electropollution" book by Dr. Robert O. Becker.
- Dick Cavett
- "Dirty Electricity: Electrification and the Diseases of Civilization." book by Samuel Milham MD MPH

- "Do Trees Strengthen Urban Communities, Reduce Domestic Violence?" paper by By W. C. Sullivan, Ph.D. & Frances E. Kuo, Ph.D.: http://lhhl.illinois.edu/

- Dr. Dan Batcheldor

- Dr. David Carpenter

- Dr. George Crile

- Dr. Lennart Hardell

- Dr. Jacqueline McGlade

- Dr. Jim Burch: http://cpcp.sph.sc.edu/fs/burch.htm

- Dr. John Nash Ott:_ http://www.biolightgroup.com/Ott.html

- Dr. Magda Havas: http://www.magdahavas.com/

- Dr. Philip Stoddard: http://www2.fiu.edu/~stoddard/

- Dr. William B. Kouwenhoven

- Dr. William Rae: http://www.ecopolitan.com/dr-william-rae

- "Earthing: The Most Important Health Discovery Ever?" book by Clinton Ober, Stephen T. Sinatra MD, and Martin Zucker.

- "Electrocution of America: Is Your Utility Company Out to Kill You?" book by Russ Allen

- "Electromagnetic Fields: A Consumer's Guide to the Issue and How to Protect Ourselves" book by B. Blake Levitt.

- Elizabeth Kelly: http://electromagneticsafety.org/

- EMFields: http://www.emfields.org/
- EMFnews.org: http://www.emfnews.org/
- "Exploring the Spectrum: The Effects of Natural and Artificial Light on Living Organisms." film by Dr. John Nash Ott.
- "Gasland" and "Gasland Part 2" films by Josh Fox. http://www.gaslandthemovie.com/
- George Carin
- Google Maps: http://maps.google.com
- "Health and Light: The Extraordinary Study That Shows How Light Affects Your Health and Emotional Well Being." book by Dr. John Nash Ott.
- Henry Barton
- Henry Ford
- Hertel
- International Agency for Research on Cancer (IARC): http://www.iarc.fr/
- Isaac Asimov
- John Cameron
- Leon Byerley: http://www.strikingimages.com/
- "Light, Radiation, and You: How to Stay Healthy." book by Dr. John Nash Ott.
- LIVESTRONG.COM: http://www.livestrong.com/
- Los Angeles Times: http://www.latimes.com/
- "Motorcycle Cancer" book by Randall Dale Chipkar.
- MSNBC: msnbc.com

- "My Ivory Cellar; [the story of time-lapse photography]." book by Dr. John Nash Ott.
- NASA: http://www.nasa.gov/
- Nation of Change: http://www.nationofchange.org/
- Nikola Tesla
- NPR: http://www.npr.org/
- Ornette Coleman
- Popular Science: http://www.popsci.com/science/article/2010-02/disconnected
- Ralph Waldo Emerson
- Robert L. Park
- Scientific American: http://www.scientificamerican.com/
- Spark Burmaster: http://www.environmental-options.info/
- "Sparking a Worldwide Energy Revolution: Social Struggles in the Transition to a Post-Petrol World" book by Kolya Abramsky
- Stetzer Electric: http://www.stetzerelectric.com/
- Suzanne Woelk
- The Stranger: http://www.thestranger.com/
- UNC Terrorism Research: http://www.unc.edu/spotlight/terrorism_research
- University of Arizona.
- Voltree Power (www.voltreepower.com)
- Wikipedia: http://www.wikipedia.org/

- World Research Foundation:
  http://www.wrf.org/
- Yahoo News: http://www.yahoo.com/

"None of us is as smart as all of us."
Eric Schmidt.

Useful Links

When researching electromagnetic radiation, I find the following sources to be very useful in developing the information:

The Center for Electrosmog Prevention has excellent information on wireless radiation health effects:

http://www.electrosmogprevention.org/

Two web sites that contain a collection of useful information about dirty electricity:

http://dirtyelectricity.ca/

http://www.dirtyelectricity.org/

Dr. Nina Pierpont is developing the health effects of wind turbines and infrasound:

http://www.windturbinesyndrome.com/

Dr. Magda Havas has a comprehensive EMI web site at:

http://www.magdahavas.com/

Dr. Samuel Milham authored "Dirty Electricity" and has a list of research papers at:

http://www.sammilham.com/

Elizabeth Kelly, Director of the Electromagnetic Safety Alliance, is tracking electromagnetic interference developments in Arizona, USA:

http://electromagneticsafety.org/

EMFacts Consultancy, founded in 1994 by Don Maisch, has produced a wide range of reports and papers dealing with various health issues related to human exposure to electromagnetic radiation.

http://www.emfacts.com/

EMFs.Info has a good listing of research papers on it:
http://www.emfs.info/

EMF News has a good listing of articles:
http://www.emfnews.org/

The Environmental Health Center-Dallas, Texas medically tests and treats human health problems including sensitivities to pollens, molds, dust, foods, chemicals, air (indoor/outdoor), water, electromagnetic sensitivity (EMF), and many more health problems as they relate to our environment.

http://www.ehcd.com/

FEB - The Swedish Association for the ElectroHyperSensitive:

http://www.feb.se/index_int.htm

Less EMF are a leading supplier in the USA of electromagnetic radiation products:

http://www.lessemf.com/

Lloyd Burrell, Author of "Beating Electrical Sensitivity – The Path to Tread", has an excellent website on electromagnetic radiation exposures:

http://www.electricsense.com/

Mast-Victims.org - A international community website for people suffering adverse health effects from mobile phone masts in the vicinity of their homes

http://www.mast-victims.org/

Powerwatch is a small non-profit independent organisation with a central role in the UK Electromagnetic Field and Microwave Radiation health debate:

http://www.powerwatch.org.uk/

Radiation Answers has numerous sources of radiation information:

http://www.radiationanswers.org/

These websites are tracking problems with radio frequency identification (RFID) systems that are now in common use:

http://chipfreeschools.com/

http://rfidinschools.com/

Safe in School is documenting electromagnetic hypersensitivity in children:

http://www.safeinschool.org/

Stetzer Electric have a list of research papers at:

http://www.stetzerelectric.com/

Many websites are documenting the rise in people who are reporting sickness around transmitting Smart/AMR/AMI utility meters and some of these are:

http://eon3emfblog.net/

http://marylandsmartmeterawareness.org/

http://michiganstopsmartmeters.com/

http://microwavechasm.org/

http://www.napervillesmartmeterawareness.org/

http://www.smartmeterdangers.org/

http://smartmeterhealthalert.org/

http://stopsmartmeters.com.au/

http://stopsmartmeters.org/

http://www.weepinitiative.org/

The World Health Organization (WHO) have an interesting EMF web site at:

http://www.who.int/peh-emf/en/

"The Internet is becoming the town square for the global village of tomorrow."

Bill Gates

Useful Contacts

AlphaLab

http://www.trifield.com/content/trifield-meter/

Trifield ® Meter measures all three types of electromagnetic field: AC magnetic field, AC electric field, and radio (including microwaves). The magnetic and electric detectors are 3-axis, making the meter easier to use than comparable 1-axis meter

3005 South 300 West

Salt Lake City

Utah 84115

USA

Telephone: (From outside US & Canada) Country Code 1 + 801-487-9492

Telephone: (From US & Canada, toll-free) 1-800-658-7030

Fax: 1-801-487-3877

Email: mail@trifield.com

Amprobe

http://www.amprobe.com/Amprobe/usen/Multimeters/Compact-Multimeters-/5XP-A.htm?PID=73047

The Amprobe 5XP-A Digital Multimeter provides superior features and accuracy in a smaller form factor.

Amprobe Headquarters

6920 Seaway Blvd

PO Box 9090

Everett, WA 98203

Tel: 1-877-AMPROBE (267-7623)

Fax: 425-446-6390

Email: info@amprobe.com

Ronk Electrical Industries

http://www.ronkelectrical.com/blocker.html

The Ronk BLOCKER is a device designed to reduce the off-site contribution to the stray voltage problem.

PO Box 160

106 E State Street

Nokomis

IL 62075-0160

USA

Phone: 217-563-8333

Toll-Free: 800-221-7665

Fax: 217-563-8336

Saelig Electronics

http://www.saelig.com/PSBEB100/PSSA002.htm

Owon PDS5022S 25Mhz color LCD oscilloscope with fast Fourier transform (FFT) function and battery pack has now been replaced by the Owon SDS6062.

Saelig Company, Inc.

1160-D2 Pittsford-Victor Road

Pittsford, NY 14534 USA

Toll-Free: (888) 7-SAELIG, (888) 772-3544

Telephone: (585) 385-1750

Fax: (585) 385-1768

Email: info@saelig.com

Stetzer Electric, Inc.

http://www.stetzerelectric.com/store/stetzerizer-microsurge-meter/

The STETZERiZER® Microsurge Meter by Graham-Stetzer is designed to separate the power line frequency to detect and respond to low level high frequency voltages caused by transients and harmonics on power lines. The level of these voltages is measured in GS (Graham-Stetzer) units and will vary with electrical equipment and loads. This device is recommended for use in conjunction with original STETZERiZER® filters. The STETZERiZER® Microsurge Meter was specifically designed as a companion to the STETZERiZER® Filters. The meter measures the level of harmful electromagnetic "energy" present, and its primary use is to guide effective STETZERiZER® Filter installation.

520 West Broadway Street

P.O. Box 25 Blair

WI 54616

 USA

Phone: +1 (608) 989-2571

Fax: +1 (608) 989-2570

<u>Acknowledgments</u>

This book was influenced by:

- Claudia Sandoval M.S.W. for her wisdom on how trees and nature interact with human social behaviors.

- My neighbors for their understanding and assistance with my biological experiments.

- Dr. John Nash Ott for his extensive research into health, light, and radiation. His lasting legacy of publications was a wonderful gift to the next generation:

  - My Ivory Cellar; [the story of time-lapse photography].

  - Health and Light: The Extraordinary Study That Shows How Light Affects Your Health and Emotional Well Being.

  - Light, Radiation, and You: How to Stay Healthy.

  - Color and Light: Their Effects on Plants, Animals and People.

  - Exploring the Spectrum: The Effects of Natural and Artificial Light on Living Organisms.

- The numerous people and companies who are referenced in this book that have worked diligently to bring the important science of environmental health to the masses.

"Help others achieve their dreams and you will achieve yours."

Les Brown

About the Author

Steven started his career at one of the largest university research and teaching hospitals in Europe. Working in the electrical engineering group, he obtained a Bachelors with Honors in Electrical and Electronic Engineering. Human health was a strong draw and he moved into the biomedical team, serving the regions hospitals. During this time he developed a fascination for human illness and disease and the causes of it, many of which were not understood.

He joined the Isaac Newton Group of Telescopes in 1999 and went to live in La Palma. La Palma is part of the Canary Islands, governed by Spain. During this time he worked with the leading European astronomers and developed his astronomical and optics skills. He became fluent in Spanish and their culture.

In 2001 he became a Chartered Electrical Engineer and joined the W. M. Keck Observatory in Hawaii. This was the world's leading astronomical facility and home to the world's two largest segmented mirror telescopes. Steven developed segmented optics and interferometry skills while working alongside world leading astronomers. During this time Steven constructed his own off-grid solar and wind powered home in the last of the traditional Hawaiian fishing villages in Miloli'i, Hawaii. He learned Hawaiian Pidgin English and the Hawaiian culture during his time there.

In 2006, Steven became the Director of the MDM Observatory in Sells, Arizona, USA. Working for Columbia University and later, Dartmouth College, he developed the facility to modern standards. He learned an appreciation of the native Americans and their culture from the Tohono O'odham Nation.

In 2008, Steven joined the solar power revolution that was sweeping the USA and commissioned the largest CIGS thin film solar photovoltaic installation in the world.

A year later he commissioned the largest solar photovoltaic power plant in the USA. The system rated power was quoted as 25MW AC with over 90,500 solar modules that were mounted to 158 single-axis tracker systems in three hundred acres of land.

He went on to develop the solar photovoltaic team for a large international company.

In 2010 he started to research radiation and publish the leading books on the subject. Some of the discoveries that Steven made during his independent research are:

Human and Biological Health:

- Found the cause of cancer (incorrect human environmental conditions).
- Found the preventative measures for cancer (correct human environmental conditions).

- Found the primary cause of Autism and Attention Deficit Disorder (excessively filtered sunlight by low-E coated double glazed glass combined with unnatural electromagnetic radiation exposures)

- Found the preventative measures for Autism and Attention Deficit Disorder (increased outdoor sunlight exposure in a natural green environment combined with removing the unnatural electromagnetic exposures)

- Found links between solar radiation and human health issues.

- Found links between man-made electromagnetic radiation and human health issues.

- Widespread radiation sickness in modern human society from the effects of unnatural solar radiation, electromagnetic radiation and interference.

- Found that global warming, climate change and human activities may be in the process of moving the electromagnetic environmental conditions outside of what the human can survive in long term.

- Found that the natural average age of the human appears to have been unnaturally extended from 65 to 78 due to unnatural radiation exposure from human activities and changed atmospheric radiation transmission due to the effects of pollution.

- Found that the background radiation levels in the human environment have been significantly increased due to the widespread adoption of large numbers of radioactive ionizing americium smoke detectors into the average home and workplace. Indeed, the Dieffenbachia plant appears to die off several months after exposure to residential Americium radiation.

- Linked breast cancer to disturbances in the Earth's natural magnetic field and electromagnetic radiation exposures from metal under wires.

- Developed the cause of allergies to pollen (Pollen Deficiency).

- Developed the causes of allergies to nature (Nature Deficiency).

- Developed the causes of general allergies (Environmental Poisoning).

- Found that the human has the genetics of an outdoor forest animal.

- Found that the human mind and body does not perform correctly away from the presence of a tree canopy.

- Found biological development and mutation problems in unnatural environments.

- Found that the human is genetically adapted to its latitude and longitude global location and significantly changing this may bring about illness and disease.

- Humans that have significantly changed their genetic environment have to pay special attention to keeping it within the boundaries of their genetics, otherwise general illness occurs.

- Found that environmental pollution is significantly changing the radiation levels in the human environment and this may bring about cellular development problems, sterility, illness, disease, and premature death.

- Developed the field of plant growth defects in the areas of electromagnetic interference, AC stray voltage/current/frequency, solar radiation, americium radiation, toxic light, and nighttime interference radiation.

- Linked the cause of Sick Building Syndrome (SBS) to coated double glazed glass (Low-E), artificial light, softened and demineralized water, contaminated air, sewer fumes, contaminated food, electromagnetic radiation and interference (EMR/EMI), americium radiation exposure, unnatural vibrations, and AC stray voltage/current/frequency effects.

- Developed the field of human aggression (Environmental Pollution).

- Interpreted the famous 1991 Barbury Castle crop circle: Energy systems are causing interference and the wheel is in motion for cellular growth to turn off.

- Interpreted the famous 2004 Windmill Hill crop circle: It is an engineering diagram of a sawtooth modulation continuous wave RADAR system (FM-CW) with near and far fields and the expanding electromagnetic pulse train. The center circle marks the change from near to far field.

- "Toxic Bucket" theory.

- The "Radiation Detoxification" process (Hibernation).

- Independently verified much of the work that was performed by Dr. John Nash Ott regarding health, light, and electromagnetic radiation exposures.

- Discovered that extended exposure to preserved food causes tooth decay, skin problems, stomach problems, acid reflux, indigestion, and heart burn. It is simply fixed by eating fresh organic food.

- Found that most cellular damage in the human occurs during sleep. The preventative measure for Autism, Attention Deficit Disorder (ADD), and many general human health problems may be as simple as moving into a different bedroom and turning off the electricity in there.

- Found that sewer in-line vent valves used in modern homes are leaking as they age and filling the home with sewer gas. This is a health risk and an explosion risk.

- Found that Tucson, Arizona appears to have a sonic boom infra-sound problem that may be making some of the residents sick.

- Developed the window mounted infra-sound detector.

- Found that the human indoor environment may have become toxic to cellular development due to the use of Low-E coated double glazed glass, metal furniture, energy star lighting products, electrical system harmonics, wireless radiation emissions, radioactive ionizing smoke detectors, and stray voltage/current/frequency exposures.

- Discovered that the Dieffenbachia plant will grow normally when it is in a biologically toxic electromagnetic interference environment when its roots are connected to one terminal of a 1.5 volt DC battery and its stem is connected to the other terminal.

Electromagnetic Radiation:

- Found that the background radiation environment has been moved out of biologically natural levels by the adoption of wireless technologies such as television, radio, cellular communications, wireless networks, RADAR, satellites, Smart/AMR/AMI meters, and so on.

- Found that exposure to the electrical system (harmonic and dirty electricity) and certain electrical and electronic products induces depression symptoms into the human.

- Found that certain electrical and electronic system exposures are a toxin to the human and that removal of the exposures causes withdrawal symptoms to occur.

- Found that microwave and radio transmissions are causing a toxic effect to occur in the human mind and body and that by reducing the exposure causes a withdrawal reaction to occur.

- Developed information regarding electrical poisoning from anti-static devices (ASD) and grounding (earthing) systems.

- Discovered that electromagnetic radiation and interference is a stimulant to the human mind and body, just like alcohol and drugs.

- Characterized man-made electromagnetic exposure in the human body: Headaches, increased sexual desire, changed personality, aggression, and fatigue. Over exposure leads to aches and pains, general illness, arthritis, depression, dementia, mental illness, cancer, and premature death. These are documented as Radio Wave Sickness (RWS), Electromagnetic Hypersensitivity (EHS) and Chronic Fatigue Syndrome (CFS) in the medical community.

- Found that the human mating and fertility cycle is triggered by electromagnetic radiation exposure from seasonal electrical storms.

- Found that the modern human is overloaded on electromagnetic radiation and interference from daily exposure to it and many people are unnaturally in a constant state of sexual desire.

- Found that the rising Autism rates are almost exactly following the rising adoption of cell phone towers and cell phones, also known as wireless radiation.

- Found that the Autism rate in boys being four to five times higher than girls appears to be due to the penis and testicles acting as receivers for man-made electromagnetic radiation.

- Hypothesized that RADAR, in particular high powered weather radar, appears to be interfering with the natural systems including human health.

- Hypothesized that RADAR emissions from automatic doors may be interfering with cellular development.

- Found that radio frequency transmitting utility smart meters, automatic meter readers (AMR), and advanced metering infrastructure (AMI) are having a toxic effect on the various biological systems that are near to them. The biological harm to the human extends for at least 76 feet from some devices.

- Found that the radiation emissions from residential ionizing americium smoke detectors are retarding cellular growth in plants.

- Found that wireless radiation puts plants into a dormant state where they follow the changes in the seasons but do not actually grow or bear fruits. They become sterile and stunted. Removing the wireless radiation exposures resurrects them.

- Found that wireless radiation affects the growth and branching structure of some plants.

- Found that plants that grow tall may instead grow low to the ground when in wireless radiation fields.

- Found that some vines will not grow into areas of biologically unnatural radiation.

- Found that wireless radiation fields are patchy and unpredictable. Just moving a few inches can be the difference between a plant being healthy and it being stunted and/or deformed.

- Found that the pulsed radiation from wireless weather station sensors and wireless utility meters can really retard and deform plants that are close to them.

- Discovered that certain electromagnetic exposures deform and retard plant growth and when removed, the plant drops all of the previous deformed leaf growth and starts growing normal growth from the tips of electromagnetic exposed part of the plant. The previously exposed part of the plant stays bald.

- Discovered that certain plants in unnatural radiation fields will only grow leaves on their branch tips at the edge of the plant. The interior of the branches of the plant stay bald. This growth pattern rectifies itself when the unnatural radiation field is removed.

- Found that certain plants in biologically unnatural electromagnetic fields will turn their growth into dark green glossy leaves with no patterning. Their leaves may be much smaller than normal.

- Developed the use of the Dieffenbachia (Dumb Cane) house plant as a biologically harmful electromagnetic radiation detector.

- Found that plants deform when grown inside Faraday cages.

- Analyzed the David Blaine "Electrified" show Faraday suit and demonstrated that it may possibly damage his health, as his protective Faraday cage was poorly engineered.

- Found that the human can get intense intestinal pains within 24 hours of exposure to high electromagnetic radiation producing car ignition systems. This may be particularly an issue in compact cars, older cars, golf carts and motorbikes.

- Theorized that Female Hysteria that was extensively documented in the 1800's was actually Radio Wave Sickness (RWS) that was induced into the females from their steel hoop and crinoline skirts that were fashionable at the time. These metal skirts were acting as Faraday cages and radio receivers for the extensive high frequency electromagnetic radiation that was present at that time from the emissions of brush generators, brush motors, the DC electrical system, and natural sources that were documented by Nikola Tesla.

- Characterized heart arrhythmia as induced from the electrical system. Exposure to overhead high voltage power lines, electrical grounding systems, and close exposure to wireless radiation transmitters can induce it. It is easily cleared up by avoiding these sources.

- Developed the "Tesla coil model of biologically harmful invisible electromagnetic radiation".

- Found that Tucson, Arizona, has installed biologically toxic transmitting automatic meters readers (AMR) on its electricity, gas, and water residential utility systems and that they are making many people in the area sick.

- Found that tall metallic structures, transmitting systems and utility systems appear to have caused an atmospheric DC voltage to go missing that appears to be essential for correct cellular development.

- Found that metal coil mattresses have AC voltages on them that are proportional to the number of electrical circuits that they are near to.

- Found that metal coil mattresses are acting as an antenna for wireless energy and contain many frequencies of energy within them. This may be a health risk to the humans that sleep on them.

- Found that metal coil mattresses distort the Earth's natural magnetic field and long term exposure to them may be a human health hazard.

- Found that metal homes and metal studded homes appear to distort the Earth's natural magnetic fields and may cause long term health problems in the human.

- Found that tall metal structures act as antenna systems and have large amounts of wireless energy on them.

- Found that tall metal structures short circuit the atmospheric layers that they are in contact with to the ground.

- Found that railroads and electrical grounding systems may have short circuited entire continents.

- Theorized that Electromagnetic Hypersensitivty (EHS) that is being reported in approximately 300,000 Swedish people may partially be caused by natural electromagnetic radiation deficiency from excessively electromagnetically shielded homes and workplaces. This can occur through the use of metal siding, metal roofs, aluminum foil radiant barriers, windows that have electromagnetic screening properties, insulation that has electromagnetic shielding properties, and so on.

- Electromagnetic radiation induced mental and physical illness.

- "Extinction Energy" theory.

- "Electromagnetic Blue Sky" theory.

- "Electromagnetic Population Growth" theory.

- Found that harmonic (dirty) electricity is toxic to the human mind and body.

- Found that exposure to high voltage, high current, and high harmonic energy can interfere with the sense of smell to report burning smells to the brain that are not there. It is accompanied by insatiable thirst and intoxication symptoms.

- Found that the electrical distribution system is in the process of turning into an unlicensed wide-band radio transmitter due to a high penetration of electronic power generation systems (wind and solar) and electronic products. This may cause radio wave sickness to occur in many people.

- Found that many electrical utility poles are emitting large amounts of radio waves into the human environment. They are unlicensed wide-band radio transmitters.

- Found that utility power lines and poles have many fields around them including plasma, ion, nitrogen dioxide, ozone, electric, electrostatic, magnetic, radio, radio reflection, radio interference, solar reflection, solar interference, microwave reflection, microwave interference, ground currents, stray voltage/frequency, and so on. These fields vary with the time of day, the seasons, and the type of power generation in the area.

- Hypothesized that the utility transmission and distribution system may be acting as broadcast antenna system for 50Hz, 60Hz, and harmonic energy into the Earth's core and atmosphere.

- Found that home and workplace electrical wiring is emitting large electromagnetic fields of various types into the human environment which may lead to sickness and developmental problems in the human.

- Developed the theory that in the Air France flight 447 crash, the pilots appeared to be in a state of intoxication from the effects of excessive electromagnetic radiation (EMR) storm exposure.

- Excessive electromagnetic interference from many laptop computers.

- Found that laptop computers interfere with the Earth's local natural magnetic field.

- Excessive electromagnetic interference from many flat screen digital TV's.

- Excessive electromagnetic interference from many consumer products and toys.

- Excessive electromagnetic interference from transport systems, including cars and motorbikes.

- Electromagnetic interference from electronic power conversion systems (inverters) and the effects on human health.

- Solar photovoltaic (PV) electromagnetic interference and the effects on human health.

- Discovered street light induced sickness.

- Discovered street light electromagnetic radiation premature death clusters.

- Developed theory in the field of artificial lighting induced sickness, disease and premature death.

- Linked electromagnetic fields from electrical fuse boards and utility meters to human illness and disease.

- Developed theory in the field of power-line illness and disease.

- Developed theory in the field of human AC stray voltage/current/frequency illness and disease.

- Found that the under wires on ladies brassieres are causing voltages and frequencies to appear between them when in electromagnetic radiation fields. This may induce illness and disease into women. A similar effect occurs with metal jewelry.

- Found that metal under wires in bras appear to be magnetized and interfere with the Earth's natural magnetic field which may lead to illness and disease.

- Found that conductive flooring, such as tile, may be electrified with AC voltage and may induce illness and disease into the human.

- Found that the water systems of homes and offices may be electrified with AC voltage and may induce illness and disease into the human.

- Found that toilet water can be electrified by stray voltage/current/frequency which may make the human slowly get sick and affect mental functioning.

- Found that the utility electrical companies should never have grounded their energized conductors into the Earth as it electrifies it.

- Found hotspots of man-made radiation within the typical American home that extended exposure makes the human fall into illness and perhaps onto disease and premature death. In babies and children, it will likely cause developmental problems such as Autism and ADD.

- Found that wireless communications systems should never have been developed as it has a toxic effect on the human mind and body.

- Hypothesized that the 50 Hz and 60 HZ utility power systems, and wireless communication systems may be affecting the Earth's magnetic field and atmosphere.

- Hypothesized that the large scale removal of trees may have affected energy flows between the core of the Earth and the atmosphere and may have impacted the Earth's magnetic field and atmosphere.

- Hypothesized that the mining of metals and concentrating them into the cities may have affected the Earth's natural magnetic field and atmosphere.

- Found that the electrical utility grounding system has shorted out the semiconductor actions of the natural ground and this may have far reaching consequences.

- Developed the "Electromagnetic Sandwich" health technique.

- Found that fatigue can be reduced by applying a small DC voltage between the soles of the feet and the wrist.

Solar Radiation and Light:

- Developed the causes of allergies to sunlight (Sunlight Deficiency, filtering, interference, and overexposure).

- Found that extensive photosynthesis effects are taking place within the human mind and body.

- Found that the human body goes deficient in both vitamin B12 and D when kept out of sunlight.

- Characterized the different human skin types and their solar radiation environment.

- Theorized that pollution water films are creating interference light and may be damaging water based life forms.

- Hypothesized that solar radiation appears to cause reduced height in adults and animals on islands due to the water reflections.

- Developed the field of "Toxic Light".

- Discovered the "Multiple-Sun" effect in mirrored buildings and reflective materials.

- Discovered the "Multiple-Shadow" effect.

- Developed theory regarding the "Cloud Effect" of atmospheric solar lensing.

- Developed theory regarding the "Turbulence Effect" of environmental solar lensing.

- Discovered the "Light Cross" optical effect and found that the "Red Rectangle Nebula" may not actually exist and may simply be an illusion created by Space. The "Light Cross" illusion may apply to similar objects in Space.

- Hypothesized that the aurora at the poles may be caused by helium and hydrogen stimulation from the Sun.

- Found that the human perception of the blue sky near to the Sun is different from the photographed blue sky during an annular solar eclipse.

- Unnaturally high levels of solar radiation in modern human society.

- Tree canopy light interference (interference green light).

- Water light interference (reflection, lensing, refraction, diffraction, and interference).

- Light modification by plants.

- Radiation suppression by nature.

- Developed "Nighttime interference radiation" theory.

- Developed "Atmospheric energy interference" theory for solar radiation.

- Satellite, airplane, and structure solar radiation interference.

- Developed the LAMB theory = Light of Alien Moons is Baneful (Alien Moons = man-made satellites, airplanes, chemical trails, smoke, pollution, water vapor, artificial lighting, glass, and so on.)

- Developed the LION theory = Light Interference Obliterates Nature.

- Developed the "Extinction wavelength of light" theory.

- Linked "Bee Colony Collapse" disorder to solar radiation, man-made satellite eclipses of the Sun, airplane, microwave, radio, and power line interference effects.

- Development of scientific theory from religious scripture.

- Developed the solar photovoltaic power equations.

- Found the sources of solar photovoltaic power system overloading.

- Found that solar radiation reflections from smooth Low-E float glass causes doubled plant growth rates and that the reflection from rippled acrylic privacy windows triples plant growth rates.

- Found that staring at the blue sky induces insomnia into the human.

- Found that late afternoon sunbathing induces insomnia into the human.

- Found that the human enters into improved health when sitting facing a shady ultraviolet transmitting window daily.

- Found that the human must be able to detect the rising and falling solar radiation levels during the daytime to be in good health.

- Found that outdoor exposure to the noon peak in solar radiation is critical in human health.

- Found that artificial light sources need to be different between daytime and nighttime lighting applications. Daytime lighting needs "full spectrum" products and nighttime needs standard soft white filament products.

- Found that artificial light sources when used in daytime applications should increase and decrease brightness during the daytime to emulate natural daylight.

"All truths are easy to understand once they are discovered; the point is to discover them."

Galileo Galilei

Author Contact

I hope that you found the book informative and please let me know about any questions or comments about the book. I can be contacted through the StevenMageeBooks channel on www.youtube.com.

I am a consultant in the areas that I research and please feel free to contact me for any help or assistance.

You may find my other books useful:

Solar Photovoltaic

- **Complete Solar Photovoltaics for Residential, Commercial, and Utility Systems:** Steven Magee has combined his three top selling books on solar power systems into one edition. Complete Solar Photovoltaics will train you on solar photovoltaics and show you how to design grid connected solar photovoltaic power systems. Operations and maintenance is detailed to enable you to have a complete understanding of solar photovoltaics from start to finish.

- **Solar Photovoltaics for Consumers, Utilities, and Investors:** This book details solar photovoltaic systems for consumers, utilities and investors. This would encompass residential, commercial and utility systems that are connected to the utility grid. There is a discussion of the different technologies available for the consumer and their advantages and disadvantages. For the utilities, there is invaluable advice on planning and constructing large projects. For the investor, forward looking statements try to predict the future of solar photovoltaics.

- **Solar Photovoltaic Training for Residential, Commercial, and Utility Systems:** This book details solar photovoltaic training for those who are interested in this area and also for those who are already working in the field. This would encompass residential, commercial, and utility systems that are connected to the utility grid. It is a comprehensive overview of a rapidly growing world of solar photovoltaic power generation technology.

- **Solar Photovoltaic Design for Residential, Commercial, and Utility Systems:** This book details how to design reliable solar photovoltaic power generation systems from a residential system, progressing to a commercial system, and finishing at the largest utility power generation systems. By following the guidelines in this book and your local solar photovoltaic electrical codes, you will be able to design trouble free solar power systems that give many years of reliable operation. When designed well, solar photovoltaic power generation is an excellent source of electrical power that results in much lower electricity bills, the power company will even refund you for the excess energy generated by your system if it is large enough. Building a grid tied solar power system is a relatively easy task. Given the large amount of government and electrical utility financial incentives that are available, it is a great time to join in the solar power revolution that is taking place in the world today.

- **Solar Photovoltaic Operation and Maintenance for Residential, Commercial, and Utility Systems:** This book details how to operate and maintain residential, commercial, and utility solar photovoltaic systems that are connected to the utility grid. By following the guidelines in this book you will be able to operate and maintain solar power systems that should give many years of reliable operation. Invaluable trouble shooting advice will aid in returning your system to full operation in the event of a problem.

- **Solar Photovoltaic DC Calculations for Residential, Commercial, and Utility Systems:** This book details how to run calculations for the DC circuit of solar photovoltaic systems. This would encompass residential, commercial, and utility systems that are connected to the utility grid. It covers the range of conditions that solar photovoltaic modules are exposed to throughout the year and shows how to incorporate these into an effective DC circuit that is well designed and reliable.

- **Solar Photovoltaic Resource for Residential, Commercial, and Utility Systems:** This book is a resource of information that is used in the solar photovoltaic field. This would encompass residential, commercial, and utility systems that are connected to the utility grid. It is a comprehensive collection of notes, diagrams, pictures and charts for a rapidly growing world of solar photovoltaic power generation technology. This book is illustrated in color.

Solar

- **Solar Irradiance and Insolation for Power Systems:** This book is a resource of information that is used in the solar power generation field. This would encompass residential, commercial, and utility systems that are connected to the utility grid. It is a comprehensive collection of notes, diagrams, pictures, and charts for a rapidly growing world of solar photovoltaic power generation technology. This book is illustrated in color.

- **Solar Site Selection for Power Systems:** This book is a comprehensive collection of images, diagrams, and notes that document the effects of light and heat in the solar power generation field. This would encompass residential, commercial, and utility systems that are connected to the utility grid. This is essential information for a rapidly growing world of solar power generation technology. This book is illustrated in color.

Architecture

- **Solar Reflections for Architects, Engineers, and Human Health:** This book is a comprehensive collection of images, diagrams, and notes that document the effects of sunlight in architecture. This is essential information for architects, engineers, and the medical profession. The discovery of the "Multiple-Sun" effect in architecture is detailed and this book is illustrated in color.

Human Health

- **Solar Radiation – A Cause of Illness and Cancer?** Illness and cancers have become part of our modern culture. It has been discovered that extremely high levels of man-made solar radiation exist in modern society. Could this be the one of the causes of illness and cancers? This book examines the increase in solar radiation and applies it to human health.

- **Solar Radiation, Global Warming, and Human Disease:** This book examines the modern development of the Earth and the potential impacts on global warming and human disease. The destruction of the forests for modern agricultural use appears to have effects that are not fully understood and these are explored. Radiation deficiency and radiation overloading are investigated to see if they are factors in many illnesses and diseases.

- **Toxic Light:** Toxic Light takes a look at the light pollution that may be in your local environment and relates it to the health problems that it may cause. Light in the human environment is only just starting to be understood and something as innocent as your sunglasses may be able to make you ill! There are many examples of commonplace items in your environment that may have the ability to affect your health. Get ready for enlightenment about the most important human nutrient of light!

- **Toxic Health:** Toxic Health takes a look at the pollution that may be in your local environment and relates it to the health problems that it can cause. Pollution in the human environment is only just starting to be understood and something as innocent as light may be able to make you really ill! There are many examples of commonplace items in your environment that may have the ability to affect your health. In particular, we will investigate if modern city life is the most toxic thing of all to the modern human!

- **Toxic Electricity:** Random aches and pains? Fatigue? Headaches? Insomnia? Facial pains? Sore eyes? Irregular heartbeats? Sick kids? Relationship problems? Blotchy skin? Hot skin? Anxiety? Toxic electricity takes a look at the electrical system and asks the question: Is this one of the most toxic endeavors that humanity has ever engaged in?

Religion

- **Solar Radiation, the Book of Revelations, and the Era of Light – Part 1:** Welcome to the Era of Light! Light has long been known to be essential nourishment for the human body. We will explore the different types of light that are present on Earth and relate it to human health and nature. Light is discussed extensively in the Bible and we will see if we can associate our findings to it. Finally, we will investigate if the Industrial Revolution has created the ultimate toxin of poisonous sunlight!

Professional

- **Engineering Science and Education Journal Volume: 11, Issue: 4, Active Control Systems for Large Segmented Optical Mirrors:** A new generation of optical telescopes is on the drawing board. These will be true giants with primary mirrors having a diameter of up to 100 meters. The technology that will enable this revolution to take place was developed at the W. M. Keck Observatory in Hawaii, where the world's largest segmented mirrors are in daily use. This article looks at how the W. M. Keck Observatory proved the mirror technology that will be behind this new generation of telescopes.

You can search "Steven Magee Books" for the very latest publications.

www.youtube.com videos supporting the ideas in the books can be found by searching: StevenMageeBooks

"Life-transforming ideas have always come to me through books."

Bell Hooks

Made in the USA
Charleston, SC
07 September 2013